MARTIN HONEYS[...]

The Joy of He[...]

HOW TO SURVIVE THE SEXUAL REVOLUTION

CENTURY PUBLISHING
LONDON

Copyright © Martin Honeysett 1984
All rights reserved
First published in Great Britain in 1984 by
Century Publishing Co. Ltd.
Portland House,
12-13 Greek Street, London W1V 5LE
ISBN 0 7126 0491 X (paper)
0 7126 0490 1 (cased)
Typeset by Deltatype, Ellesmere Port
Printed in Great Britain in 1984 by
Richard Clay Ltd., The Chaucer Press, Bungay, Suffolk

We live in the age of the permissive society,

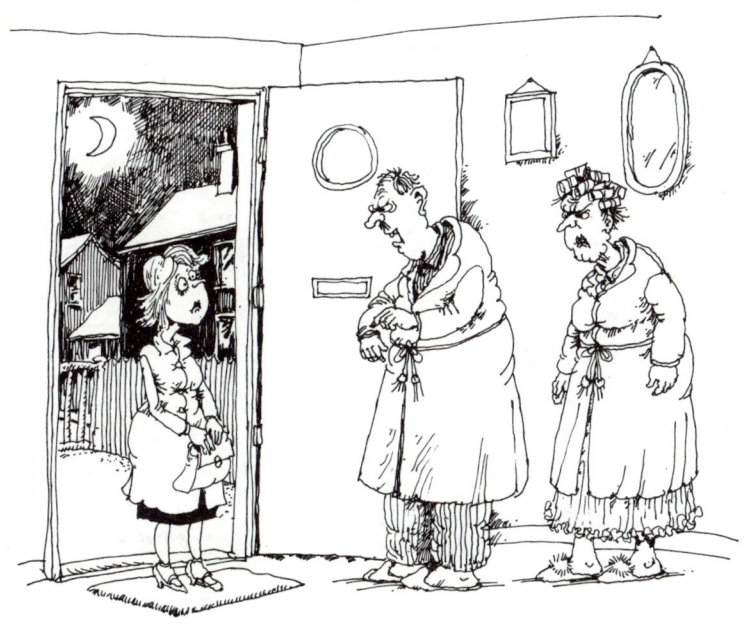

We told you to be home from the orgy by twelve!

brought about by the sexual revolution.

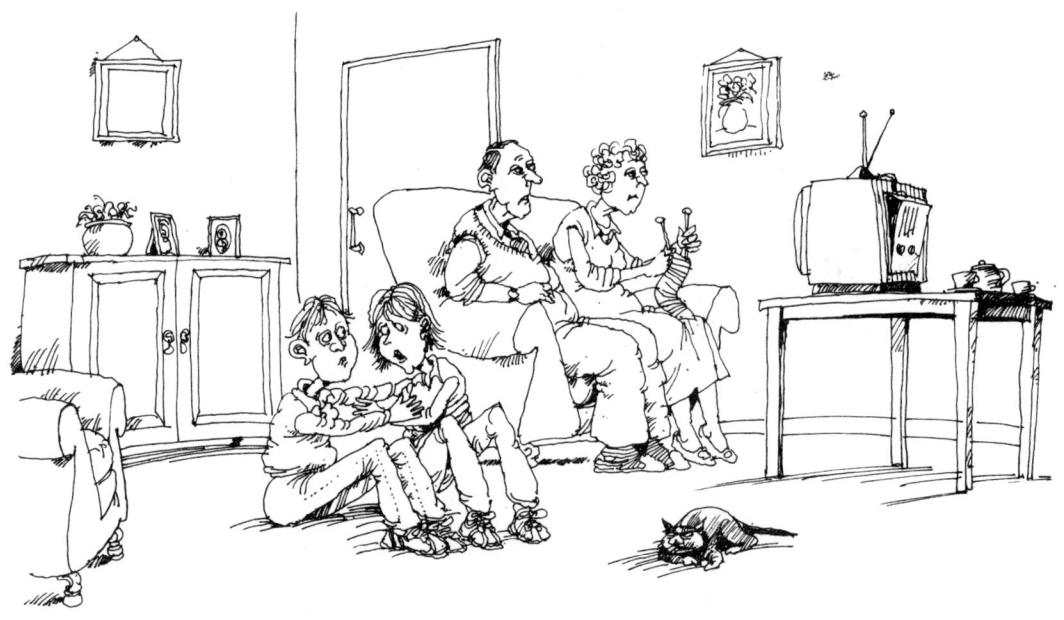

No — not in front of the parents.

A few decades ago . . .

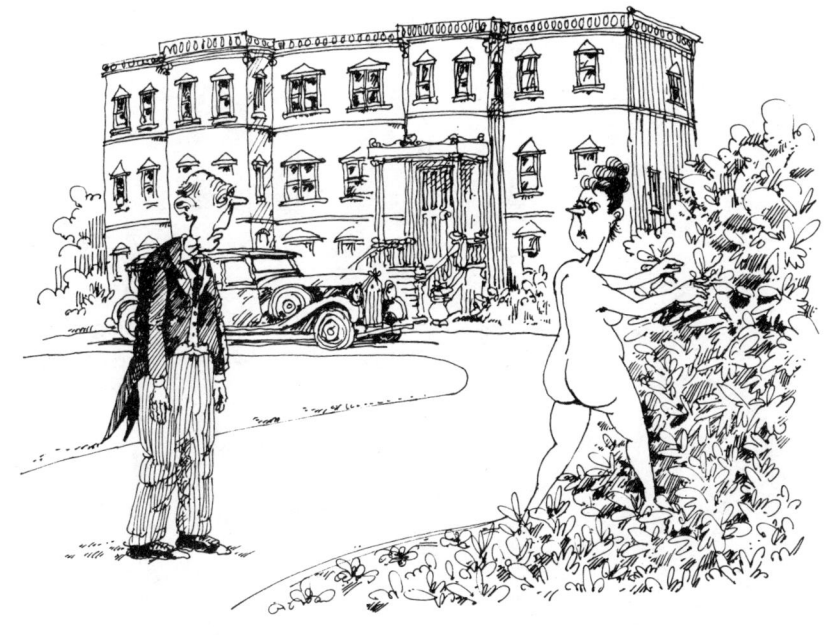

I believe it's the gardener's day off, Ma'am.

sex was a private, even furtive business . . .

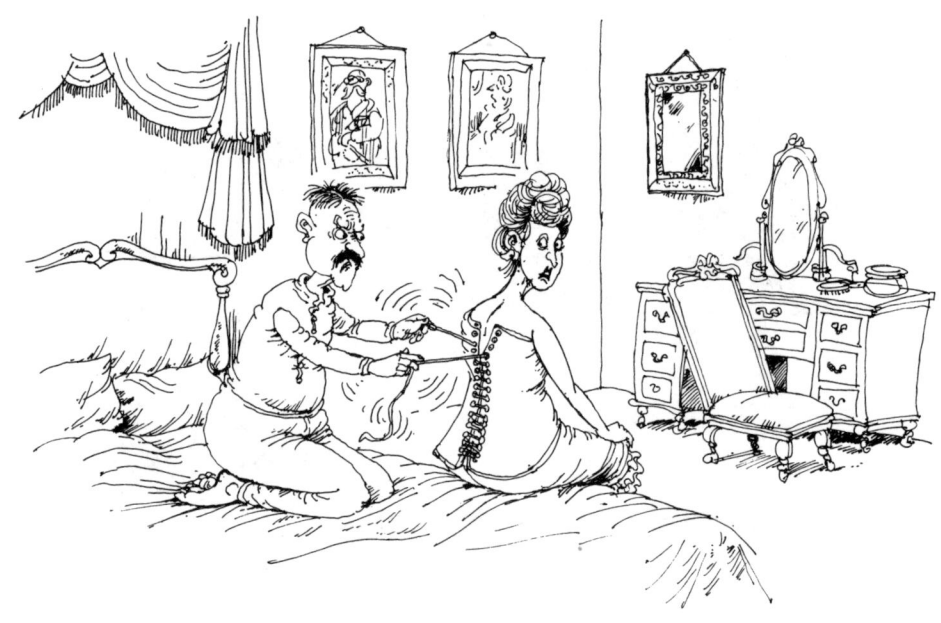

Hurry up — my husband will be back next week.

conducted behind closed doors.

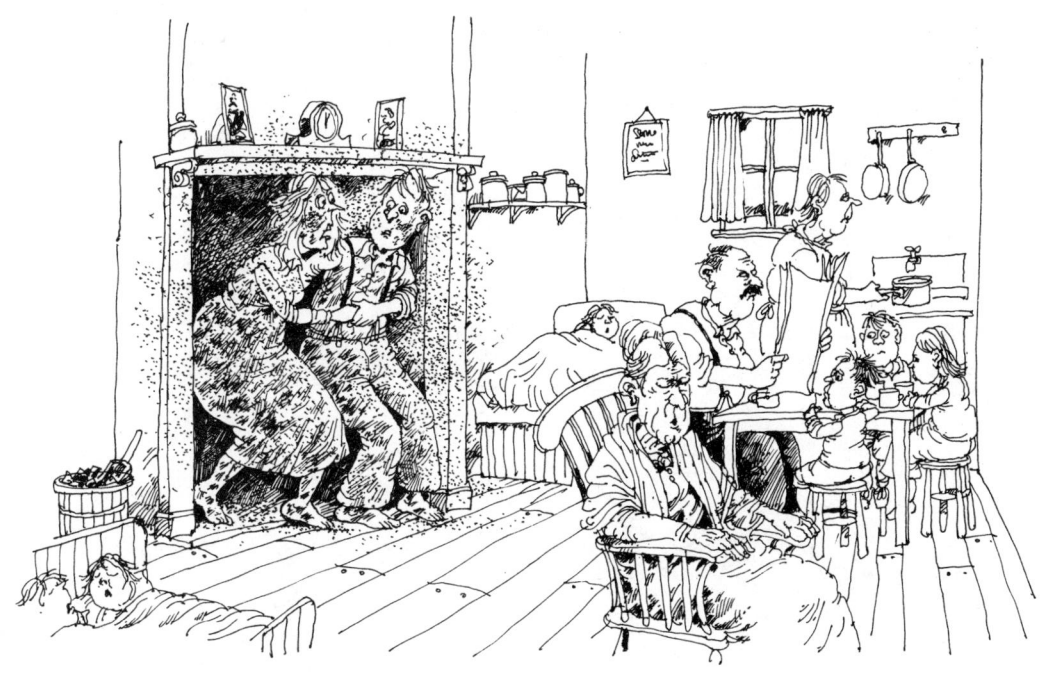

If only there were somewhere else to be alone.

The swinging '60s changed all that . . .

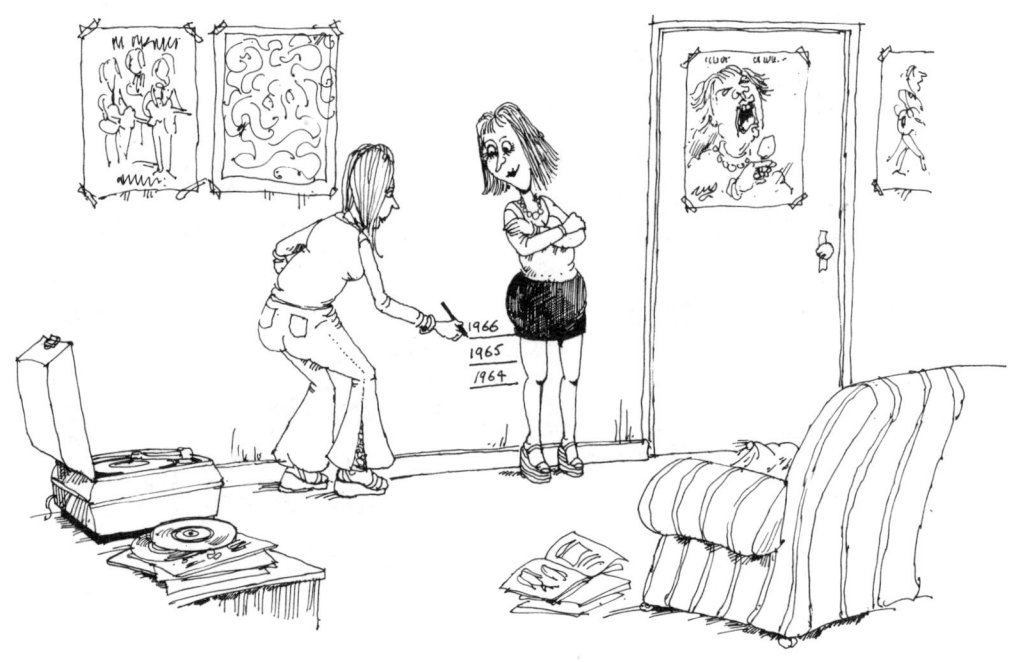

and brought sex out into the open,

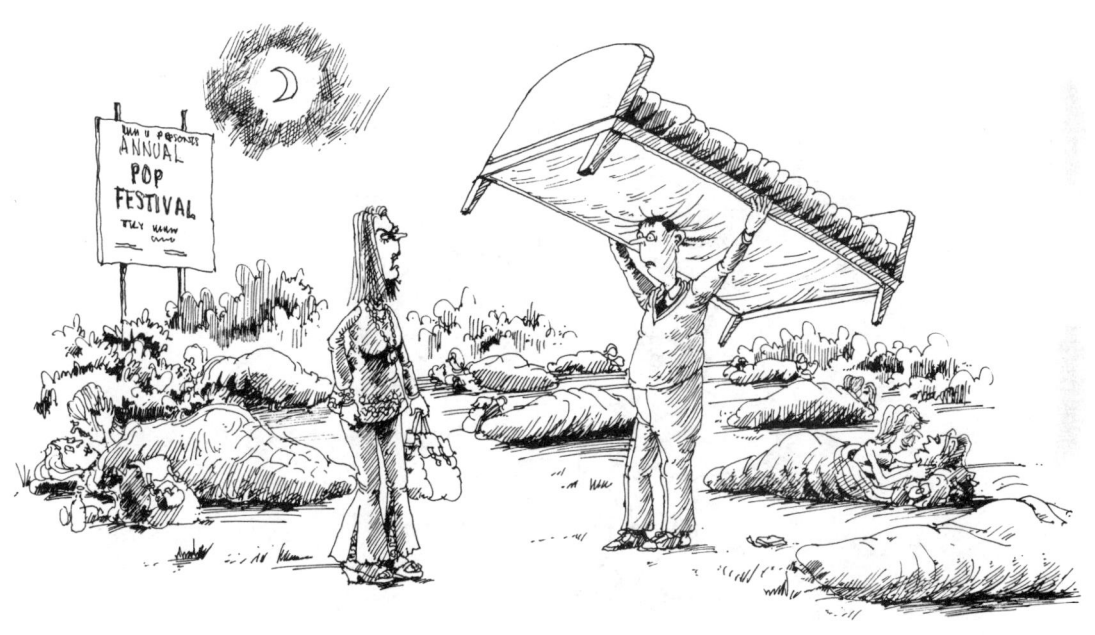

Do you have to be so square, Henry?

heralding a new era of **sexual freedom**.

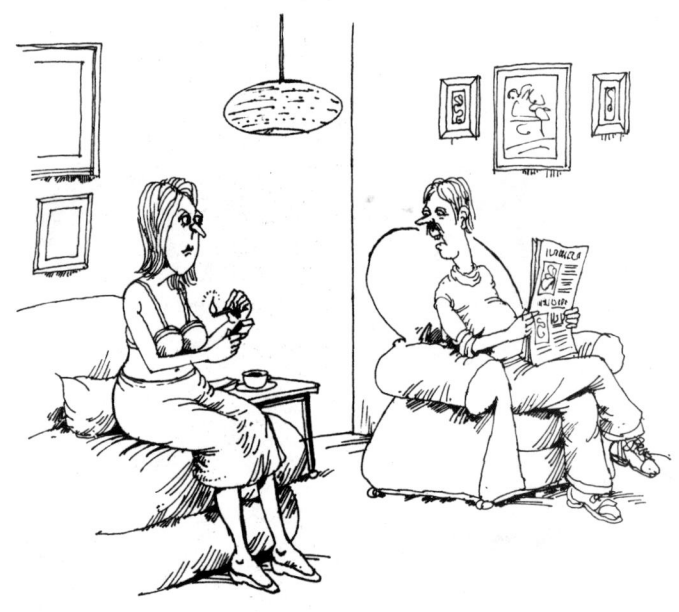

I know it's none of my business, but shouldn't you take the bra off before you burn it?

Since then, sex has been publicised . . .

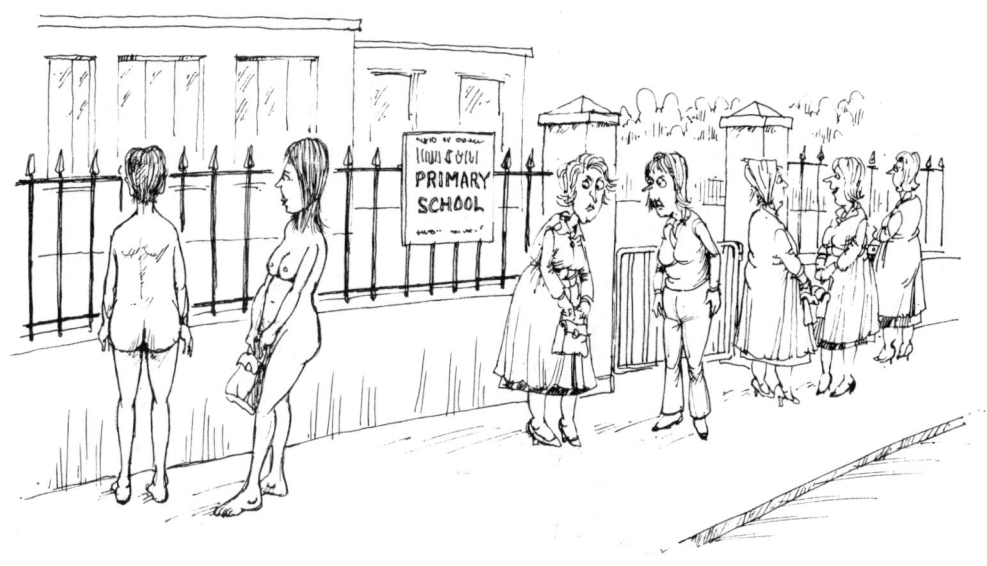

They're the sort of people who think their children ought to see them naked from time to time.

and commercialised as never before . . .

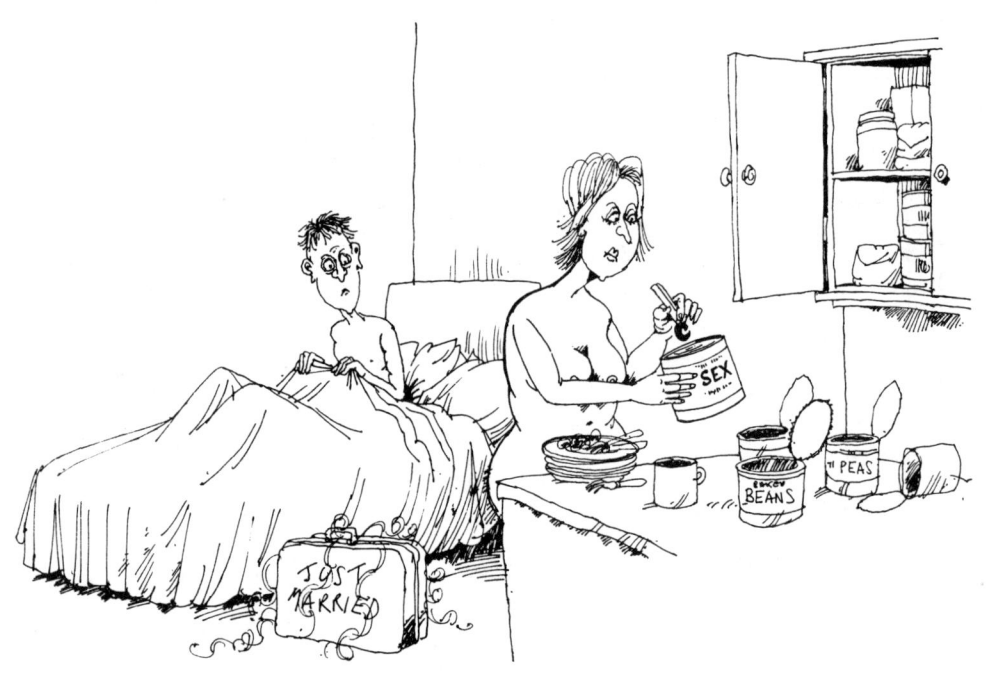

—so that today . . .

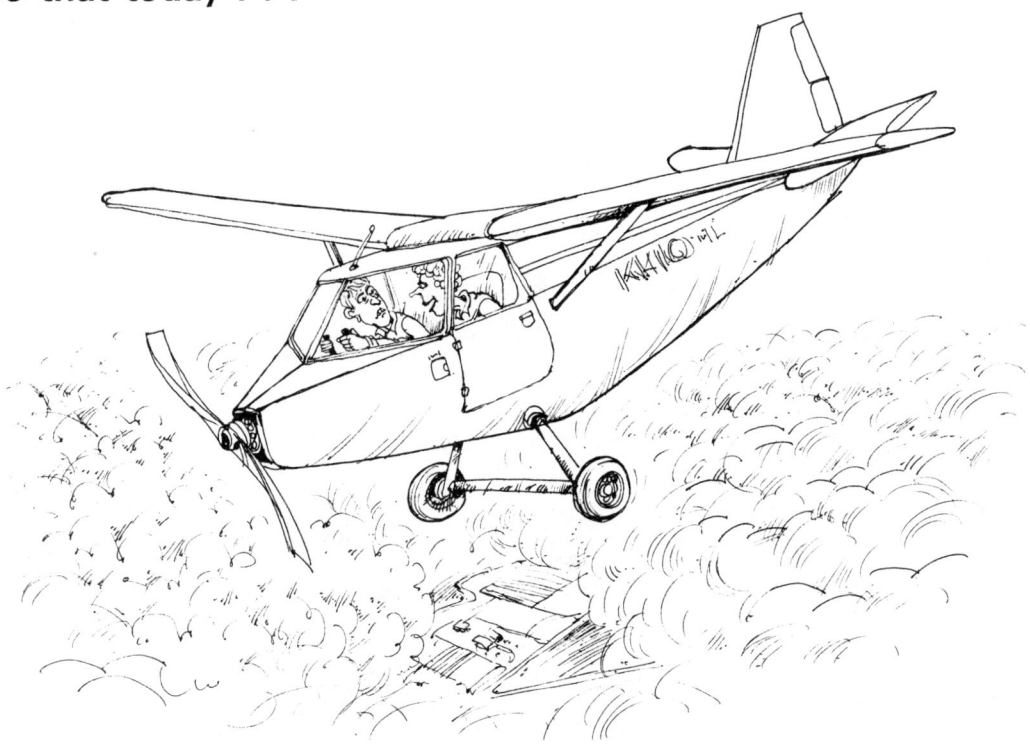

Run out of petrol! You don't expect me to fall for that old one?

we are constantly being reminded of it . . .

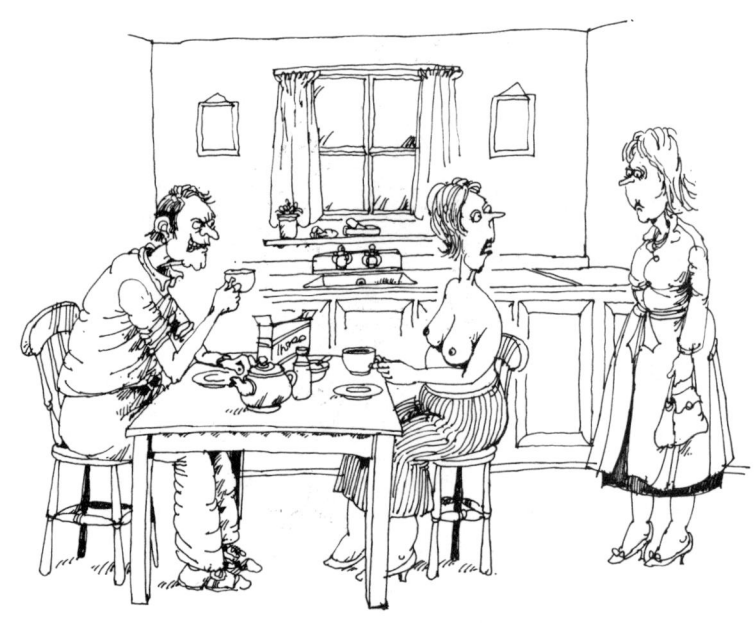

It's not the news he misses when the papers are on strike — just Page Three.

in one form or another.

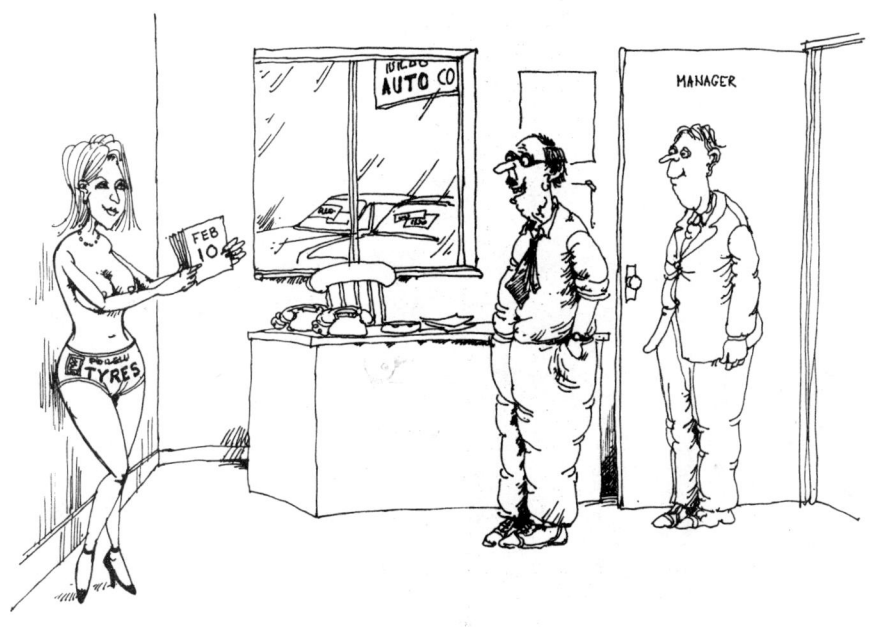

*Their calendars **get better** every year.*

Research in the '50s showed that many people were ignorant about sex,

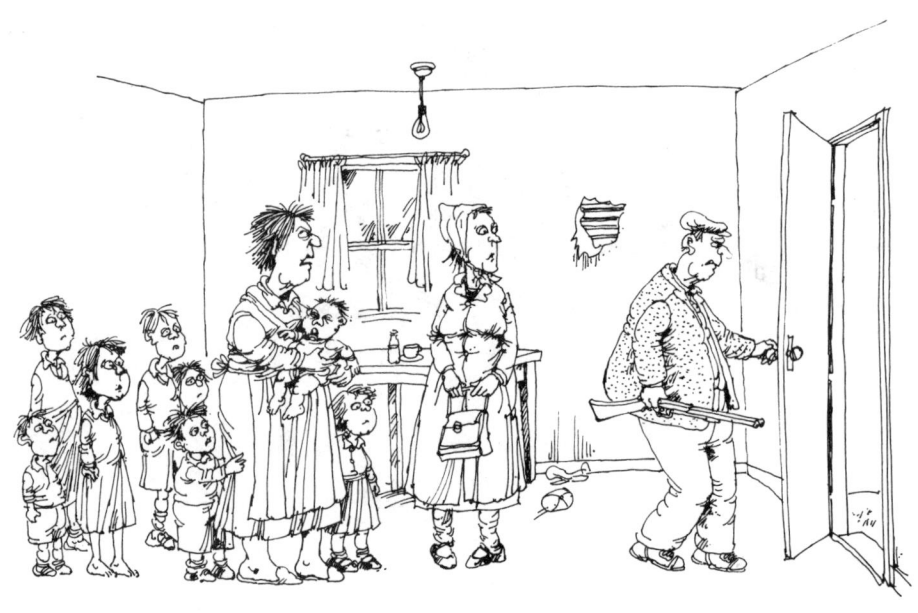

We don't want any more kids, so he's going out to shoot the stork.

and the wedding night was often their first sexual experience.

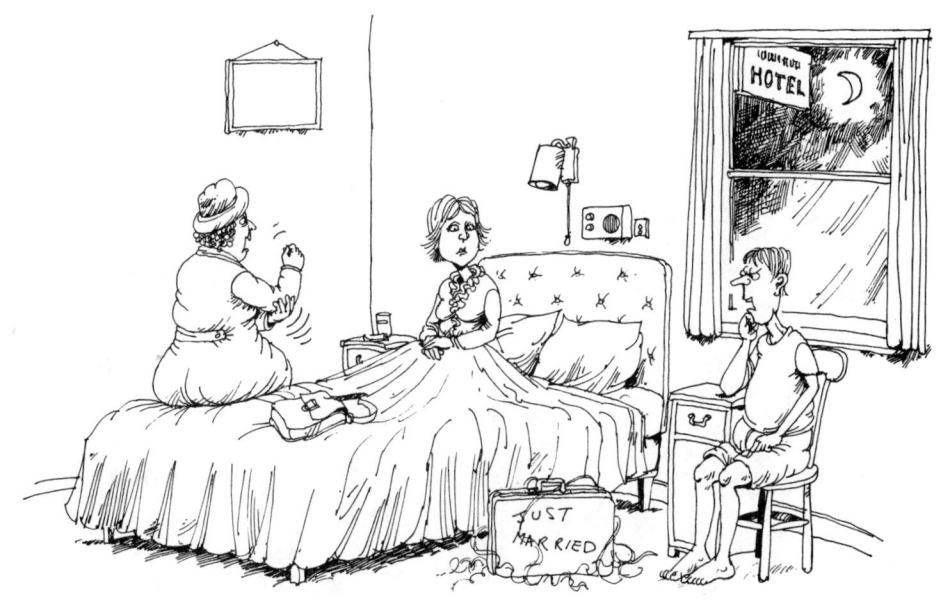

She's picked a fine time to tell you about things, I must say.

Today, thanks to all the books, magazines and films,

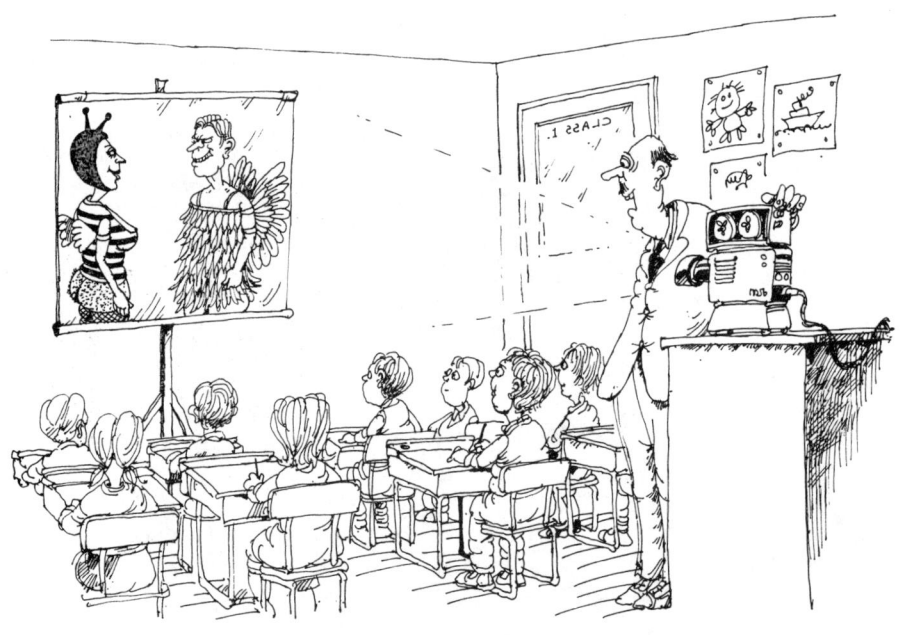

Today we're going to learn all about the birds and bees.

everyone can be an expert.

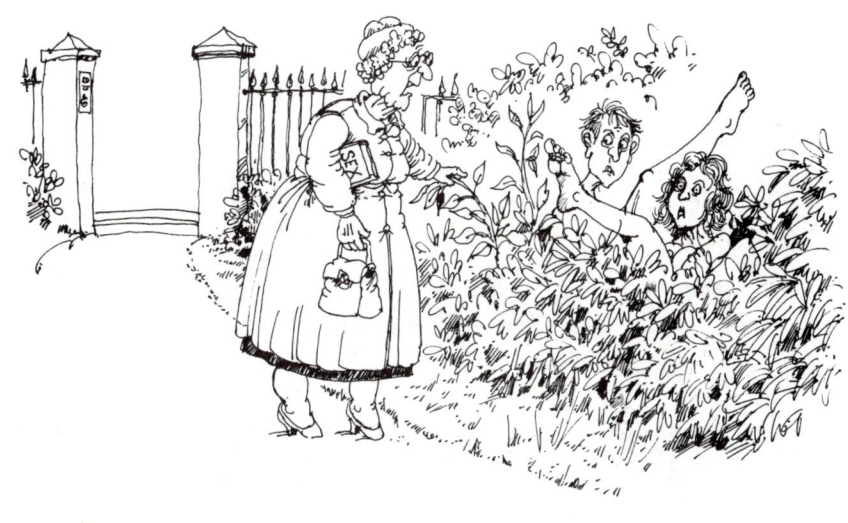

If that's supposed to be number 54, your right arm's in the wrong place.

Sex manuals have been big sellers over the last few years.

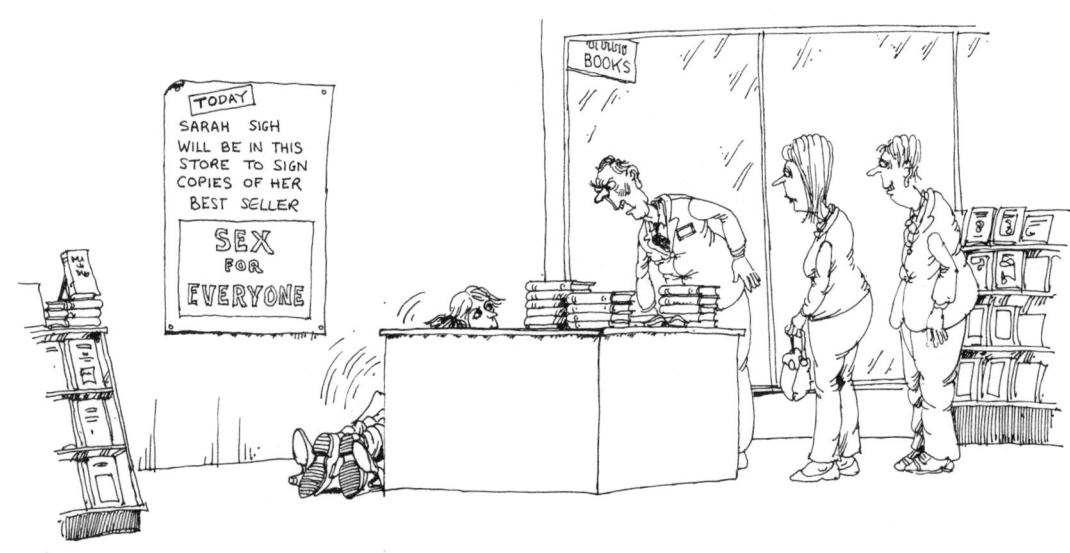

You only have to sign a copy for each customer, Miss Sigh.

They explain in detail . . .

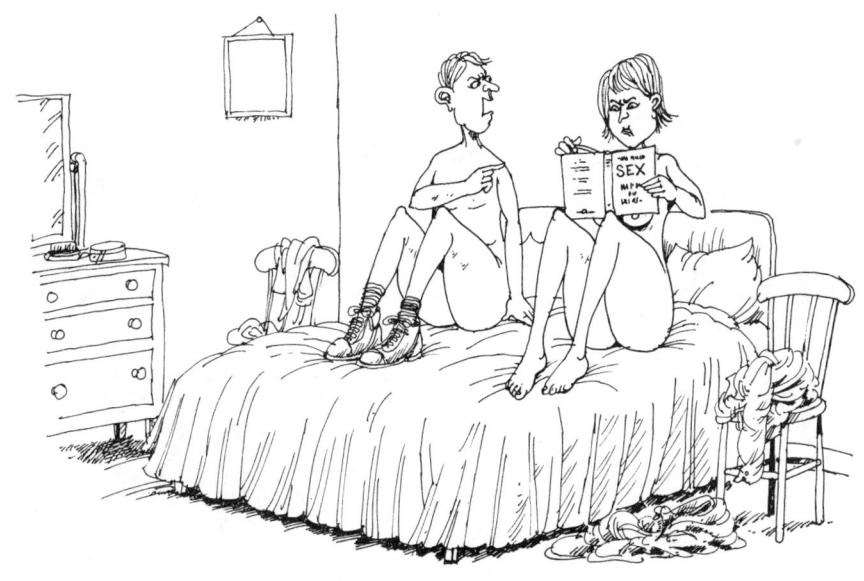

The book doesn't say anything about taking boots off.

all aspects of sex and personal relationships,

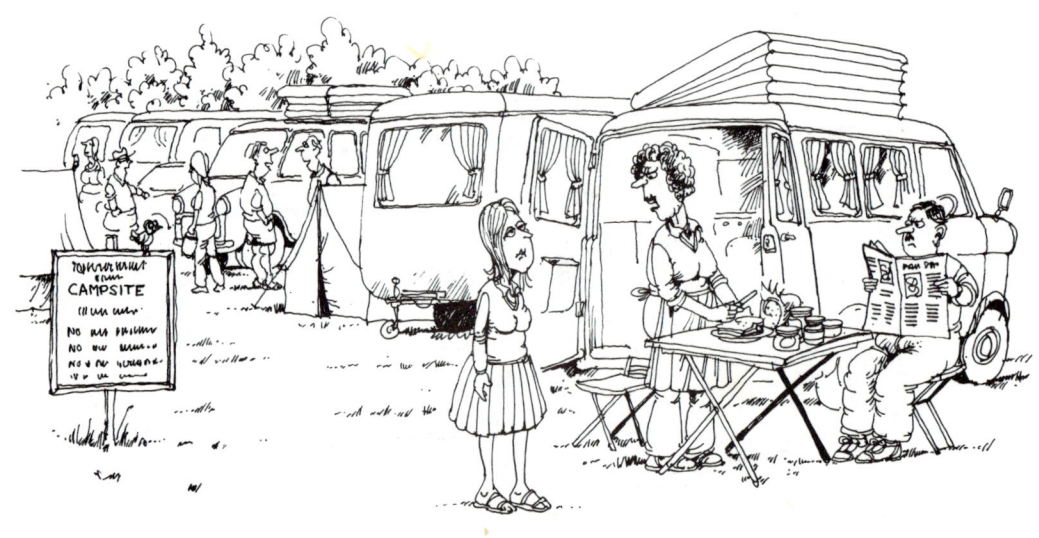

And stop telling people you've been 'sleeping around'.

exploding some of the myths that surround sex.

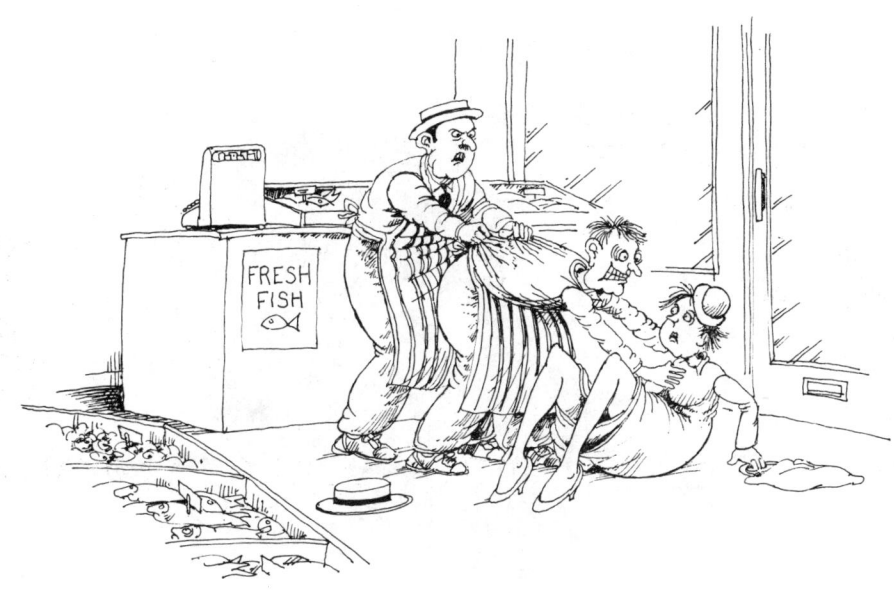

I'm sorry, Mrs Simpson — he's been at the oysters again.

You *can*, for example, get pregnant making love standing up,

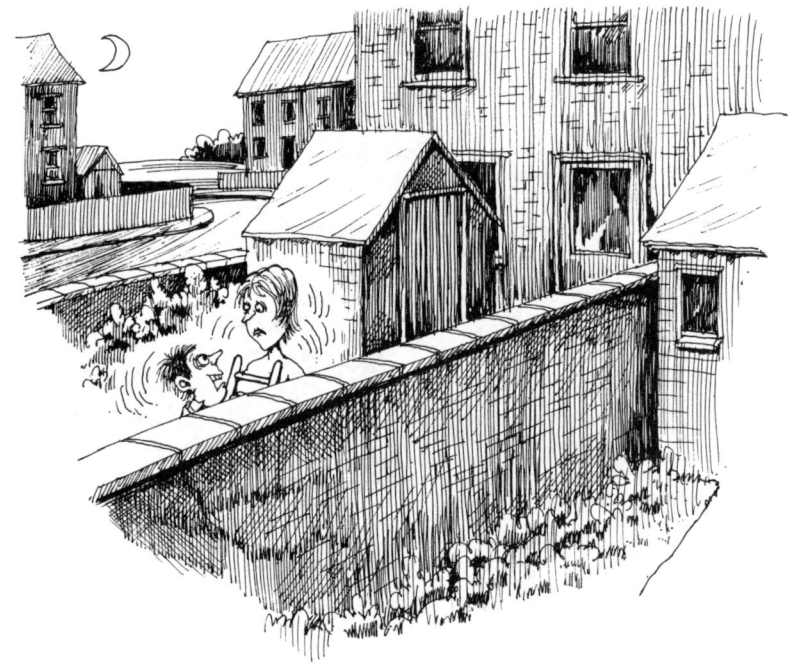

Of course it's safe — I've never fallen off the ladder yet, have I?

and size is *not* important.

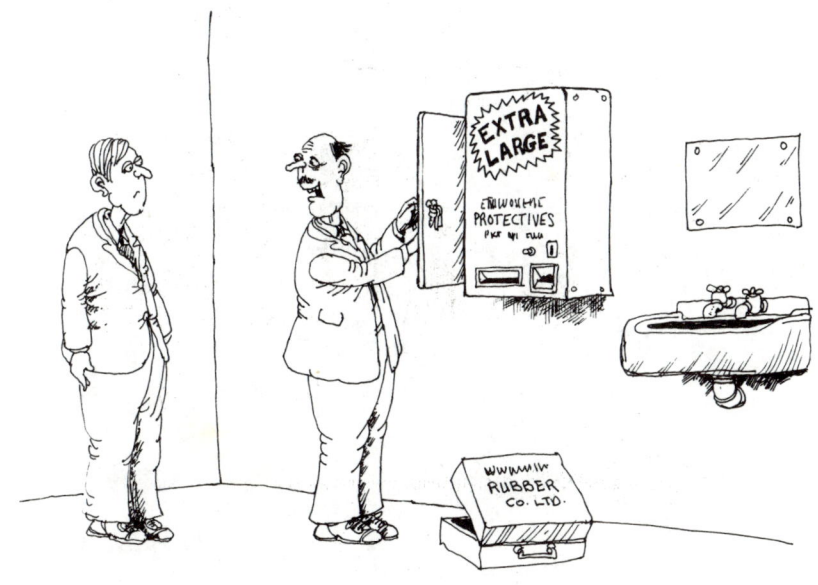

Actually they're no bigger at all, but we sell an awful lot of them.

With the aid of explicit diagrams,

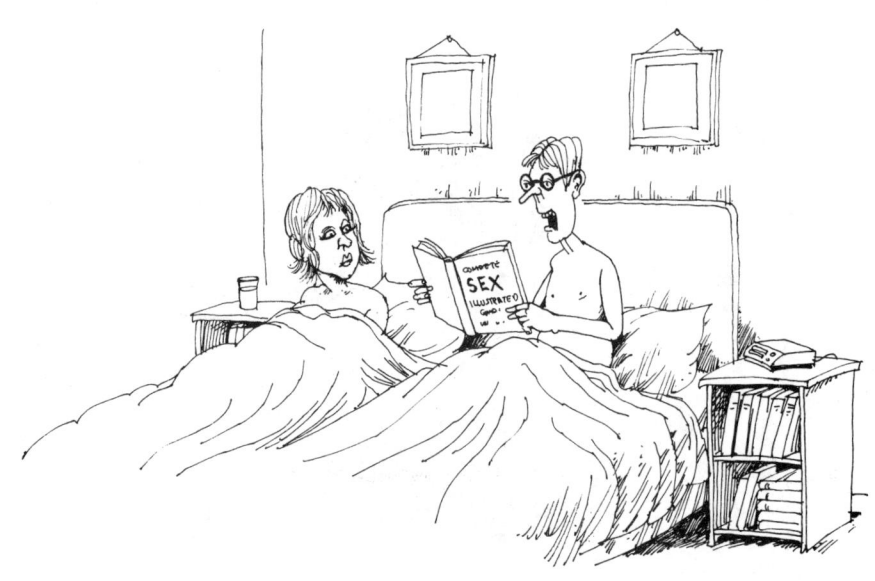

I can only read one page at a time before my glasses steam up.

we can learn about our sexual organs . . .

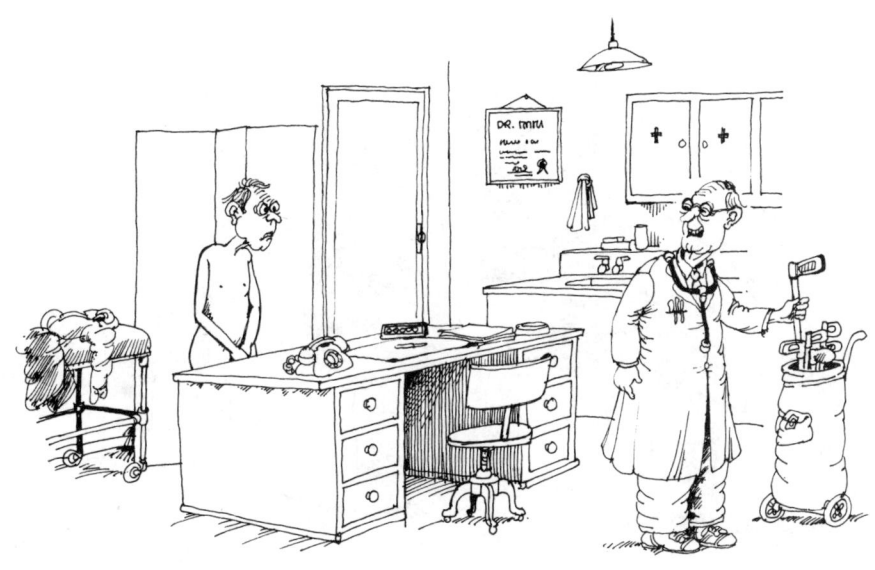

Don't worry, Mr Dobson, they won't hang half so low when I've finished with them.

and their functions.

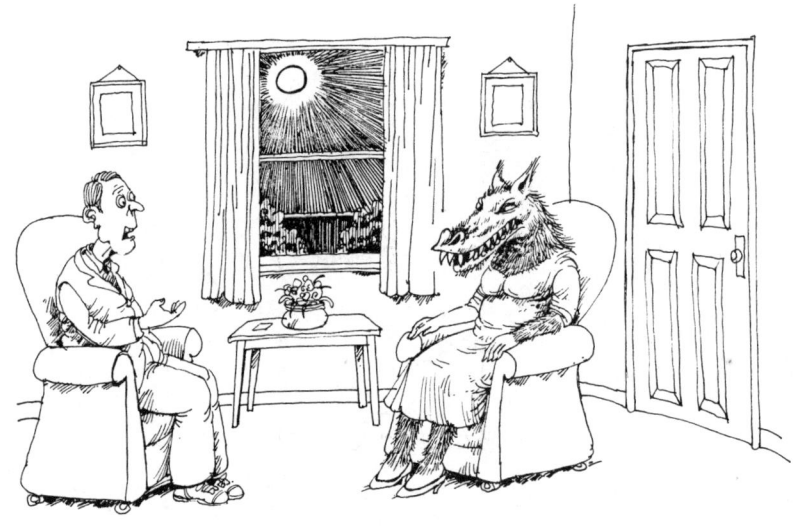

I think you ought to see someone about your periods, Doris.

They tell us how to arouse our partner with foreplay,

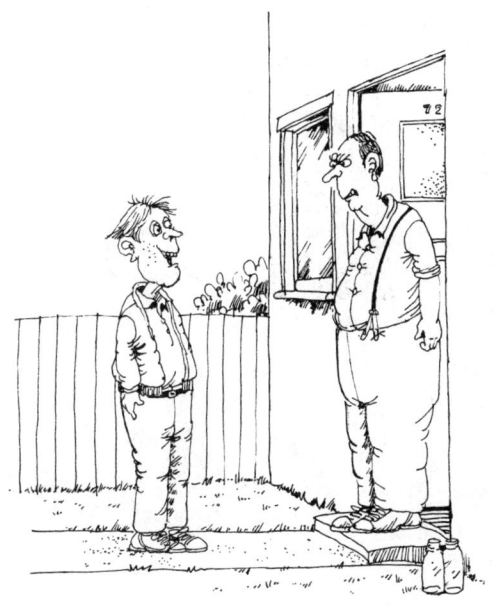

Can Jane come out to foreplay?

the art of oral love-making,

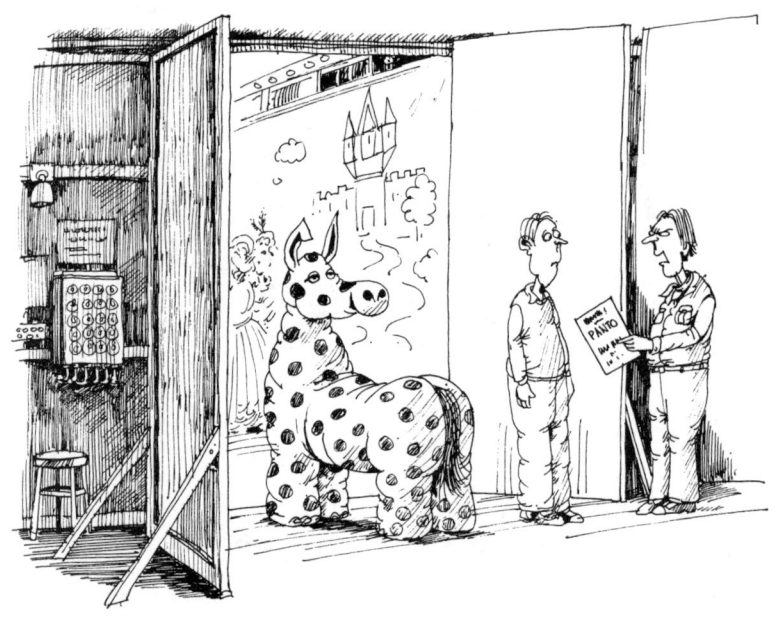

I don't care if they are man and wife, they're not going on stage like that.

and how to have intercourse . . .

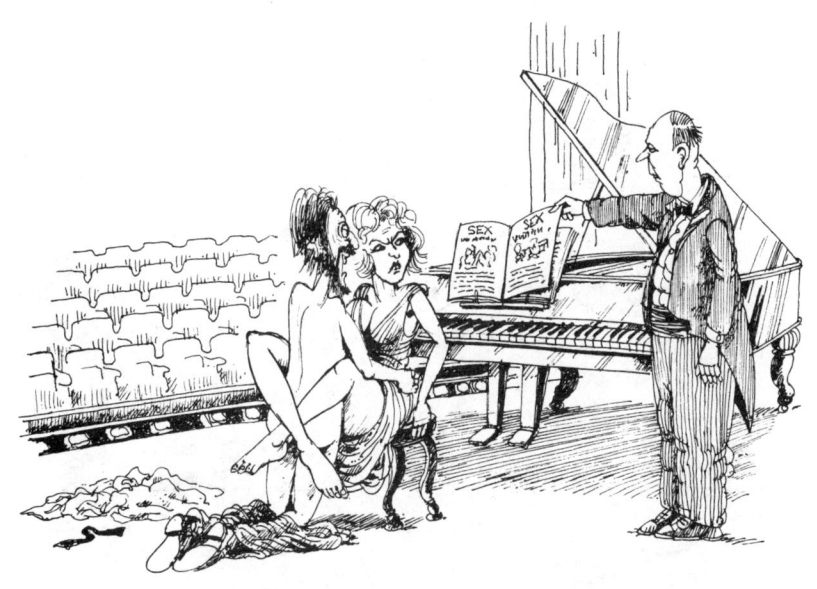

But he always turns my pages.

in any number of positions . . .

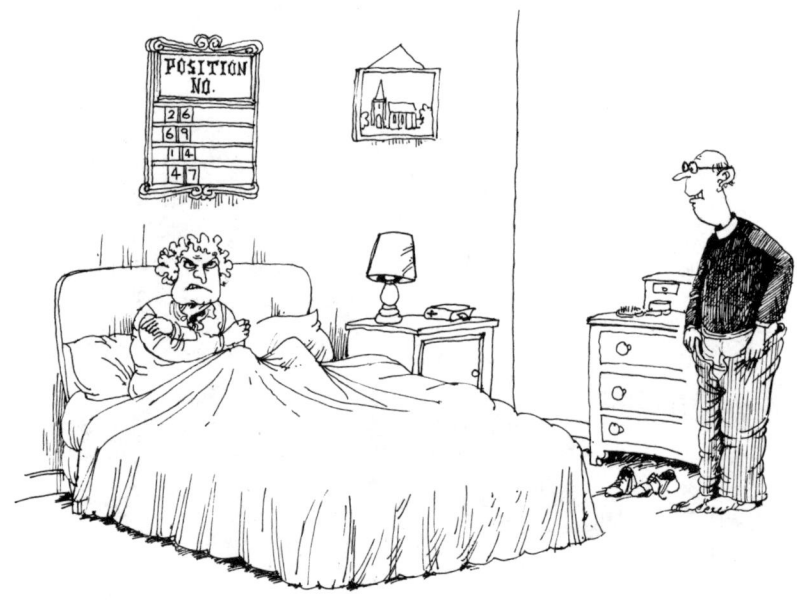

— **for the full enjoyment of both partners.**

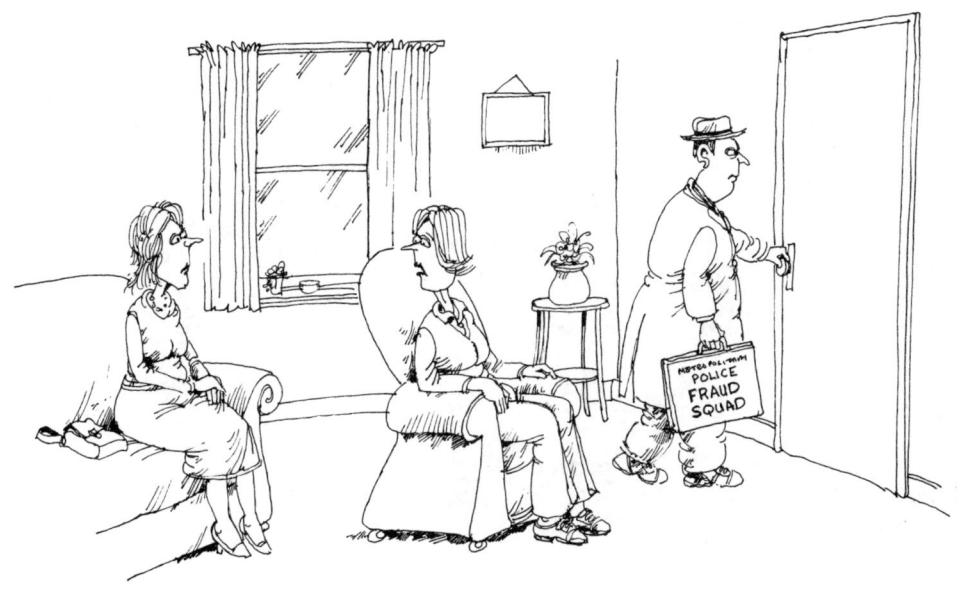

His job's affecting our love life — he knows when I fake orgasms.

They will tell you the use . . .

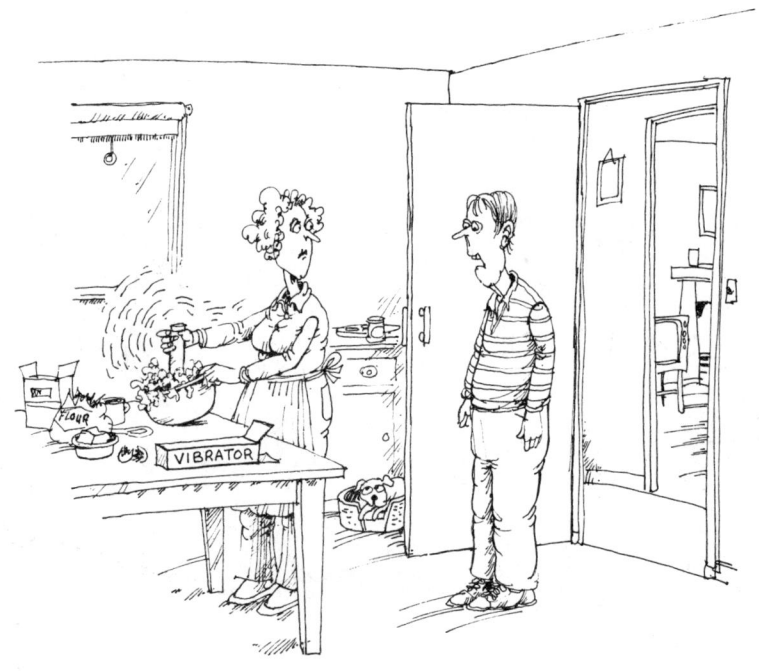

I hope you washed that after last night.

— or uselessness . . .

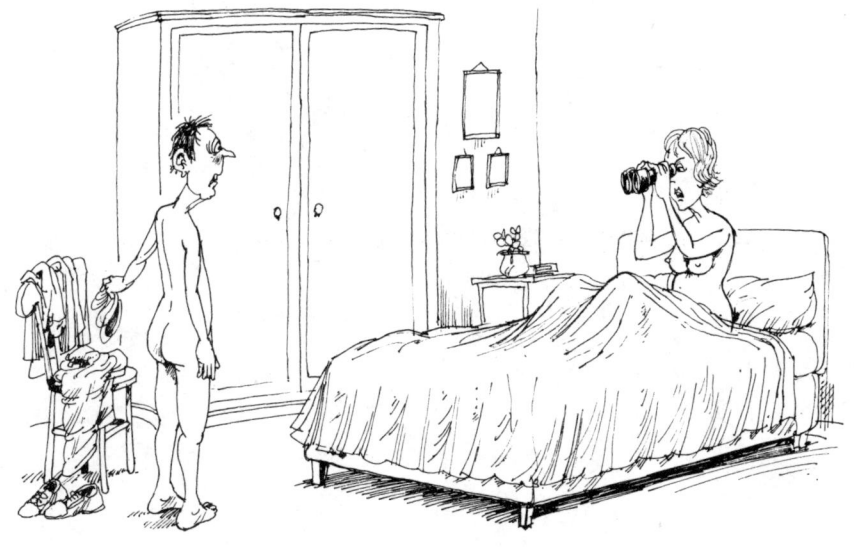

I told you that enlarging cream was a waste of time.

of stimulants and sex aids . . .

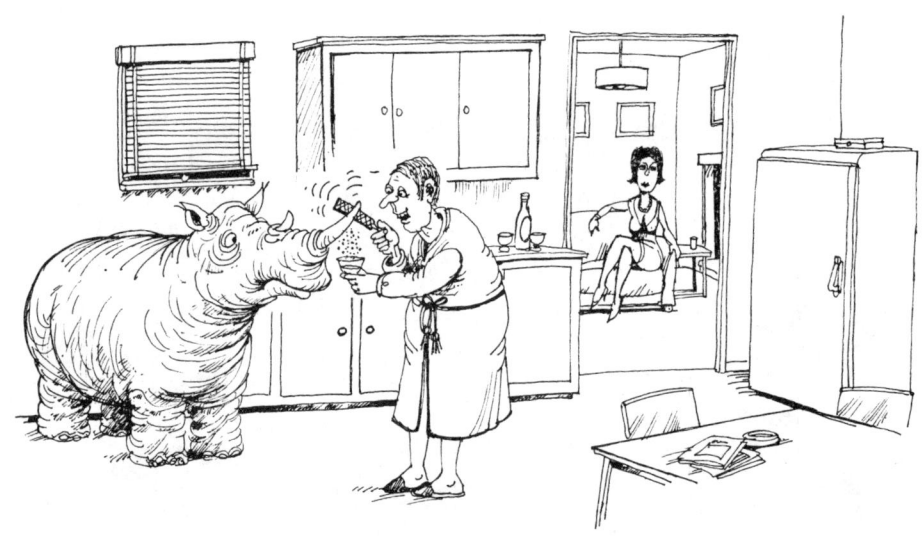

Hang on — I'll just fix myself a drink.

for those with . . .

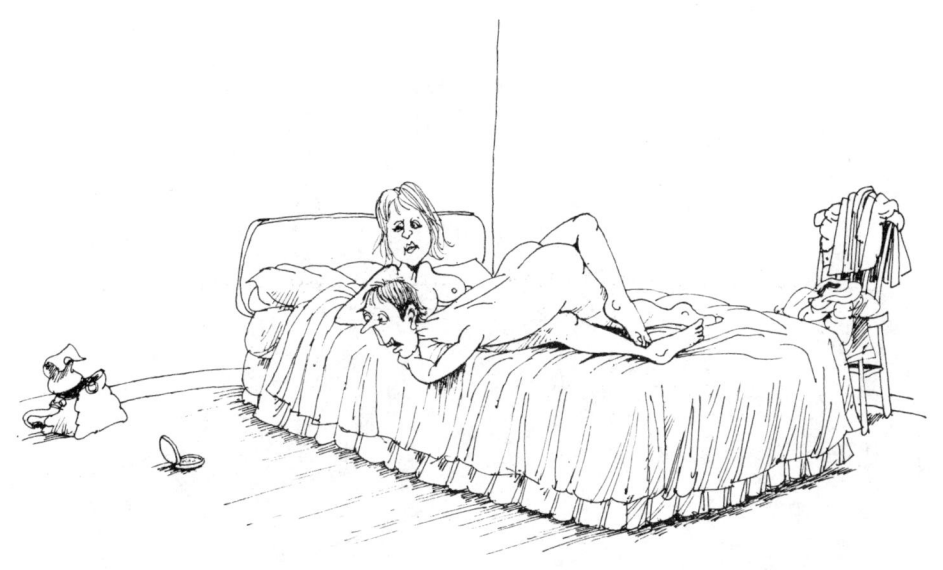

Haven't you got a bigger mirror?

or without a partner.

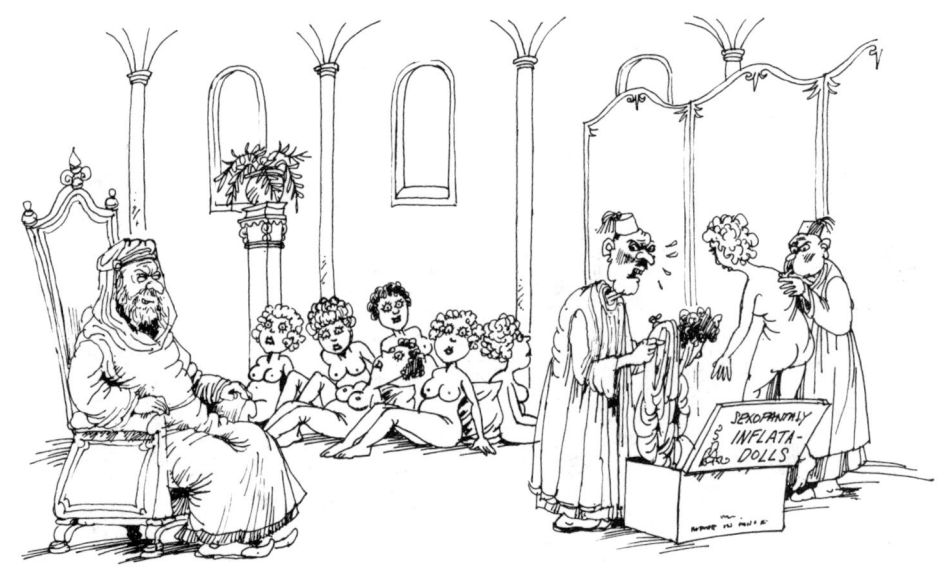

Why can't he choose one before we blow them all up?

They explain the different methods of birth control,

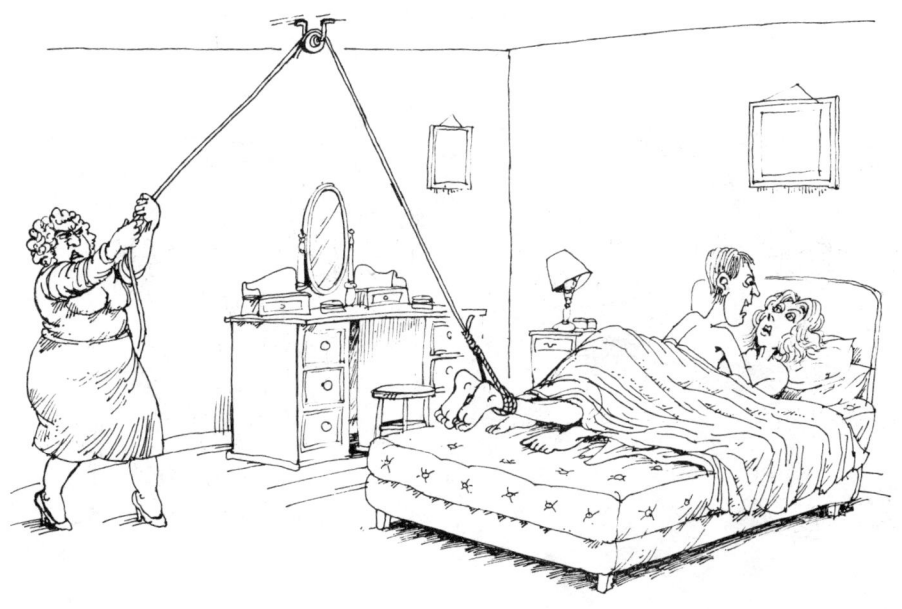

Tell your mother I'm quite capable of withdrawing on my own.

including contraceptives . . .

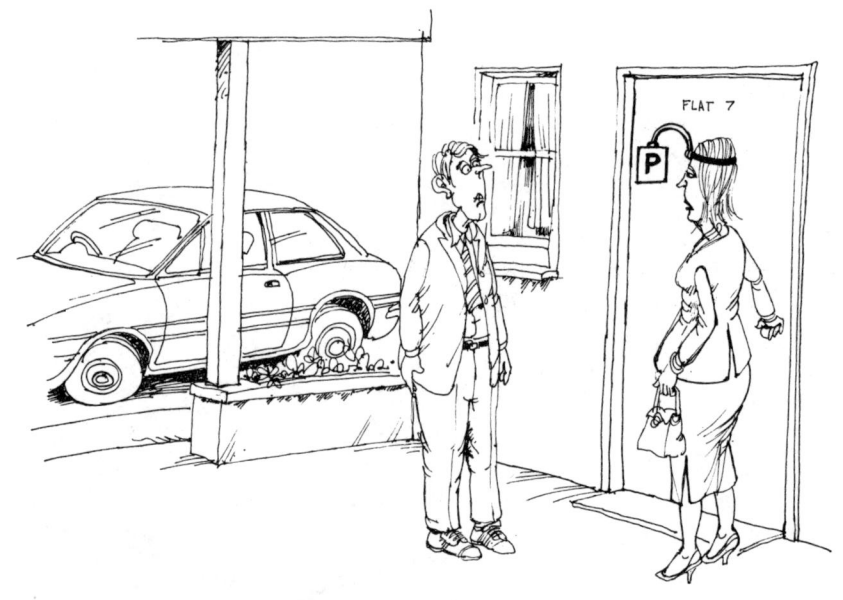

It's so I don't forget to take the Pill.

and their use . . .

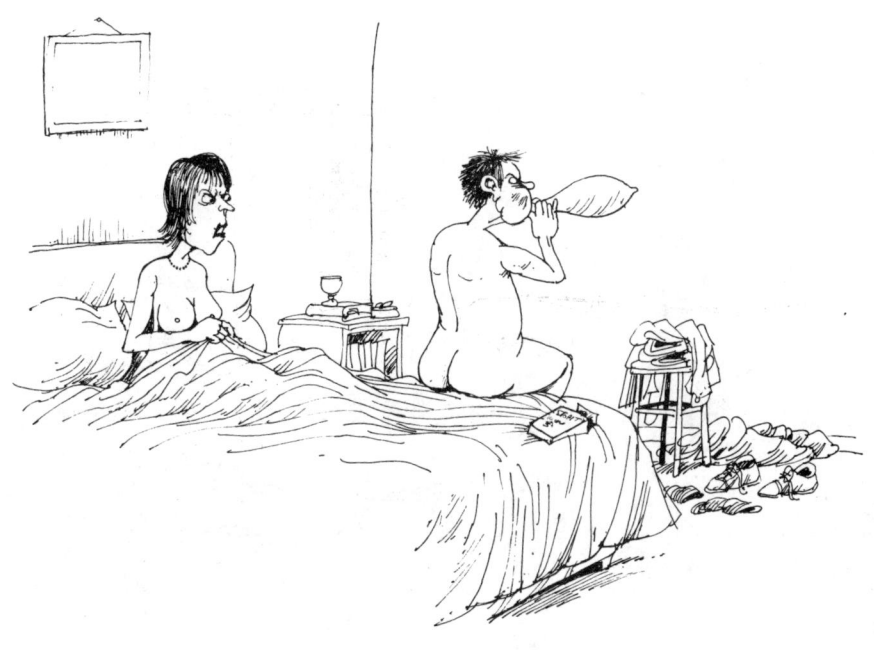

I don't care what they taught you at the Rugby Club — that's not what you're supposed to do with it.

— and what to do if you haven't used them.

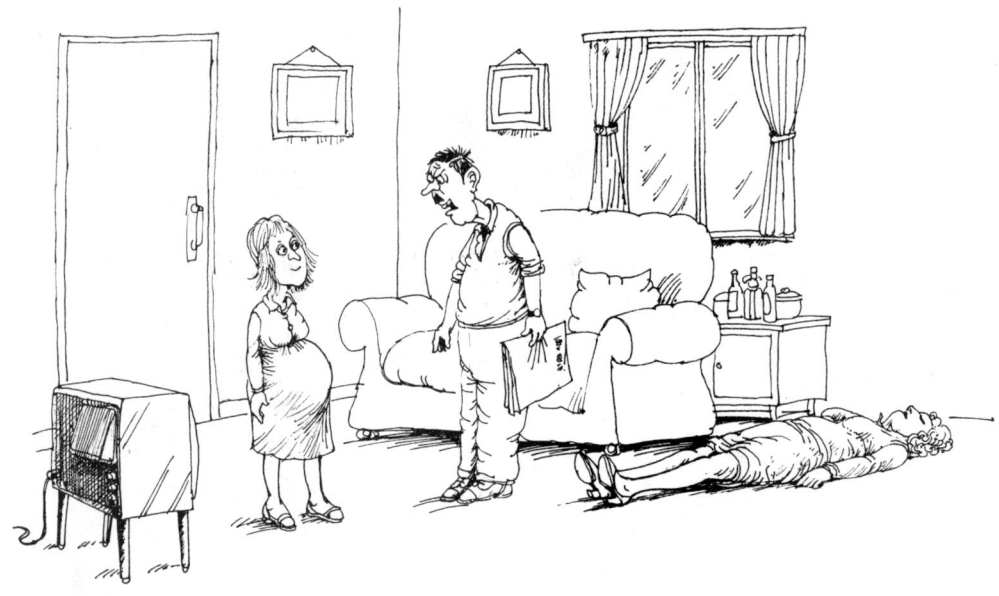

Take that cushion out — and don't play tricks like that on your mother again.

The pros and cons of vascectomy . . .

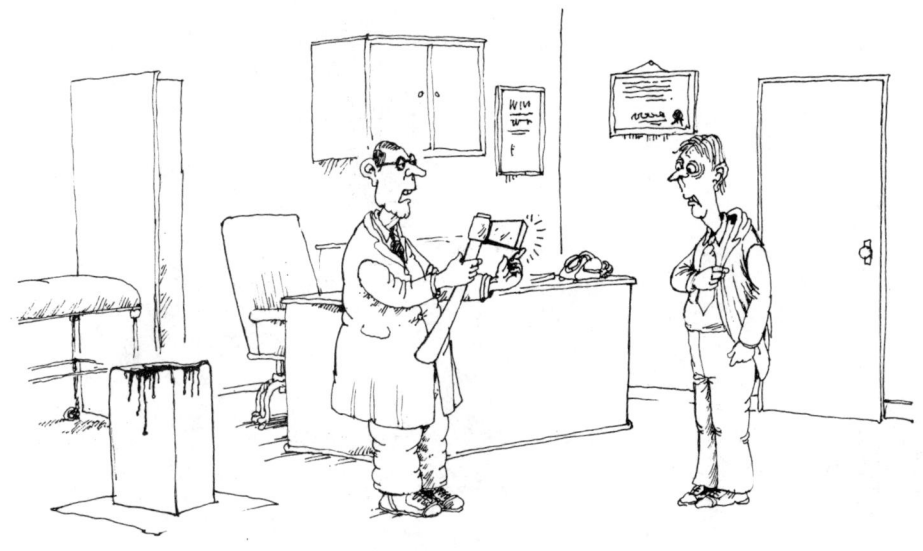

Don't worry, Mr Dobson, it's quite a simple operation.

and sterilisation are explained,

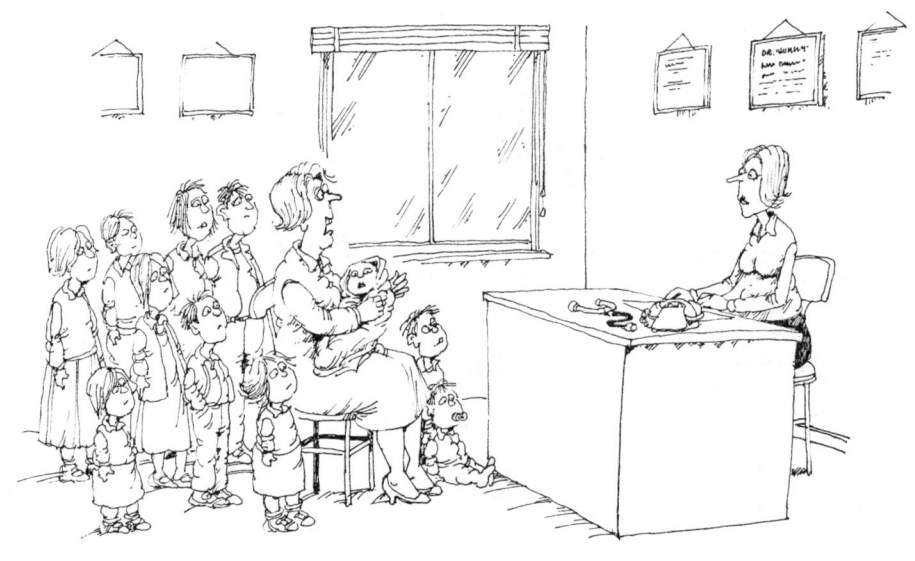

The problem is, doctor, I'm so busy with the children I haven't got time for the operation.

not to mention diseases and infections.

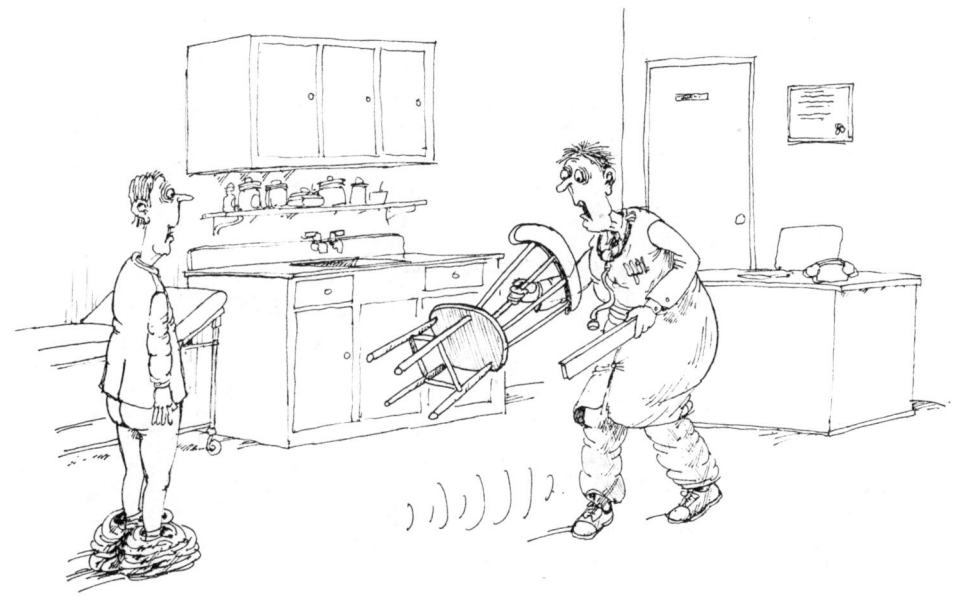

I've seen some crabs in my time, but . . .

In these days of 'anything goes' . . .

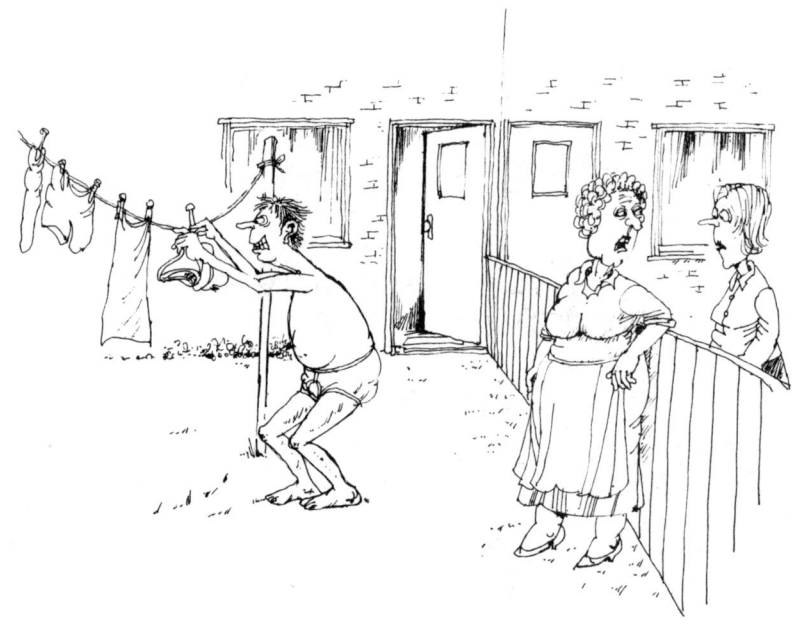

He's a lot better — now he only steals his own underwear.

— **anywhere,**

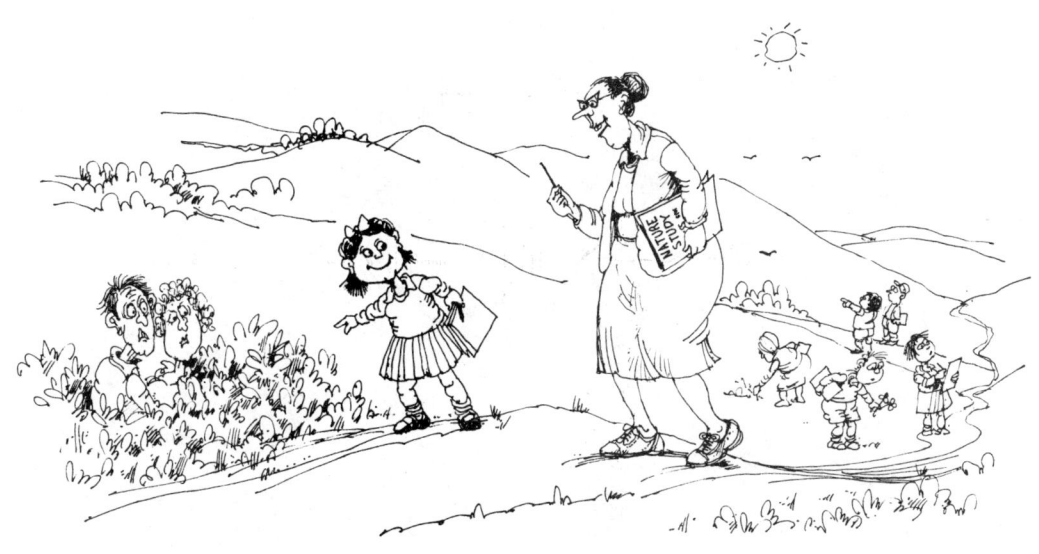

Very good, Fiona, take five points.

any time . . .

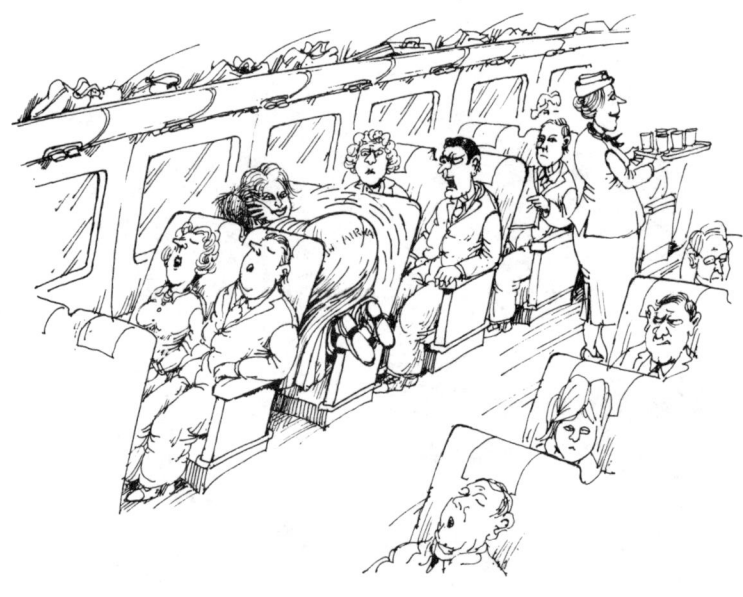

I wouldn't mind, but he's the pilot.

— **sexual practices that at one time might have been considered kinky . . .**

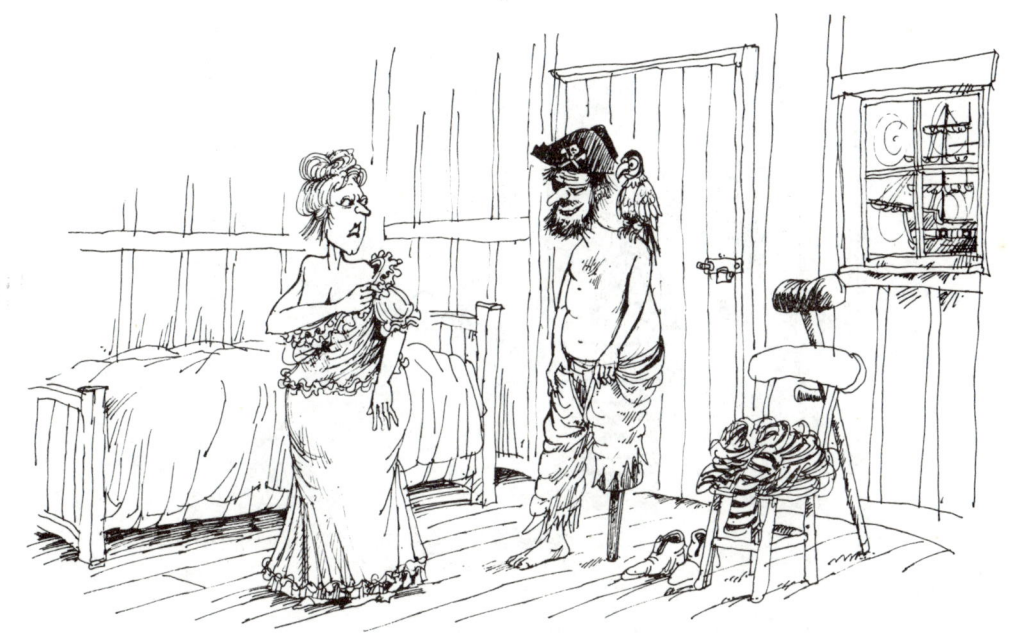

I don't mind him watching — it's his foul language I object to.

or perverted . . .

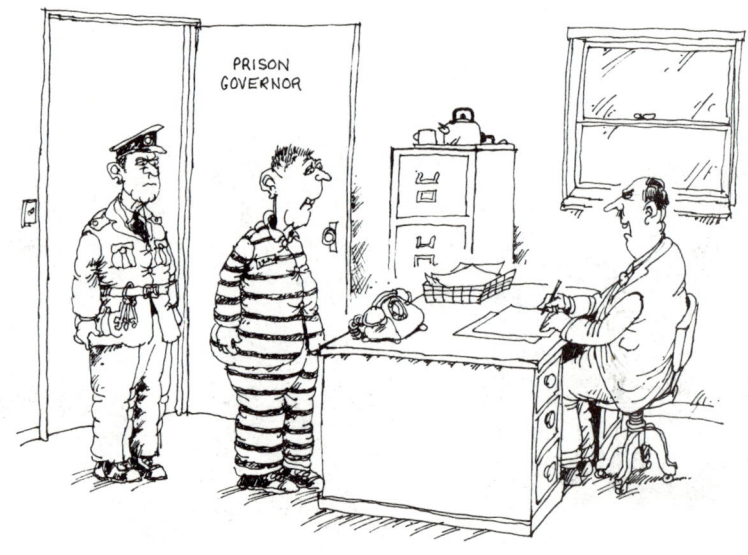

I'm afraid raping a canary is a serious offence, Jenkins.

are no longer taboo.

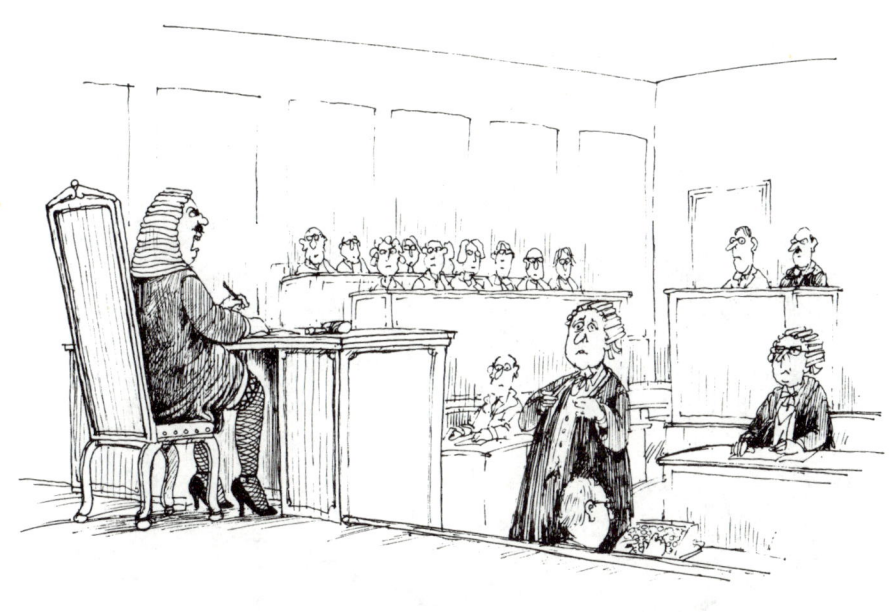

What the accused does in private is no concern of this court.

Even the more conservative sex experts will concede . . .

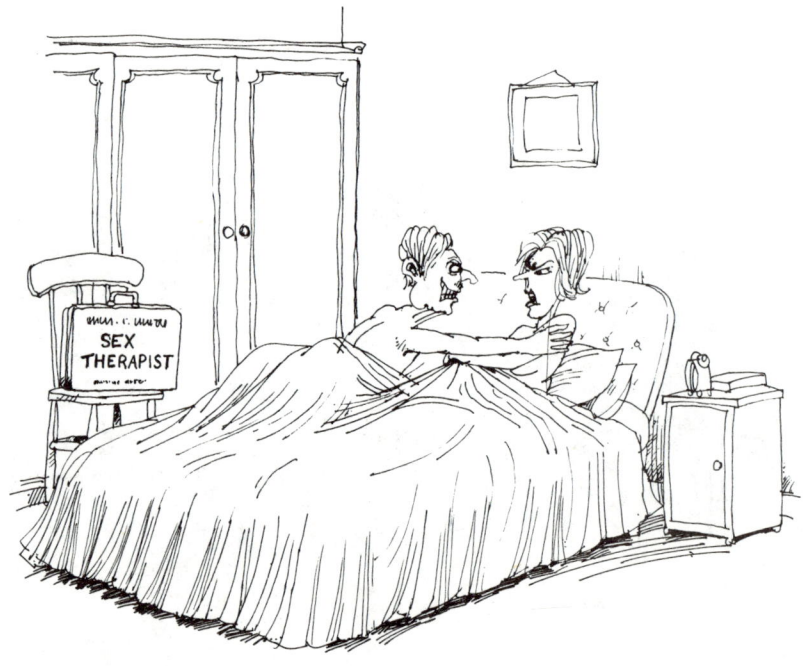

Work, work, work — that's all you ever think of.

that as long as they're not harmful,

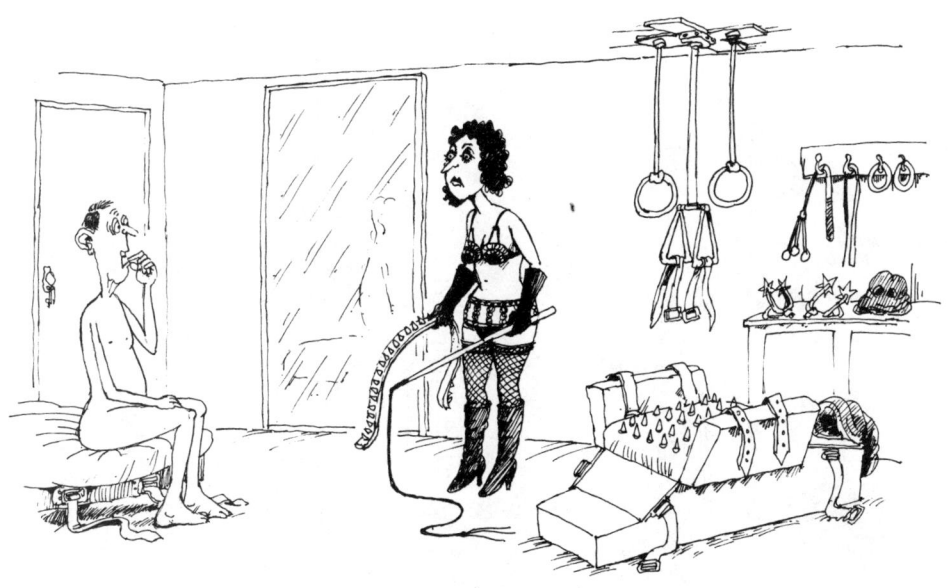

It's my first time — be gentle with me.

such practices are OK.

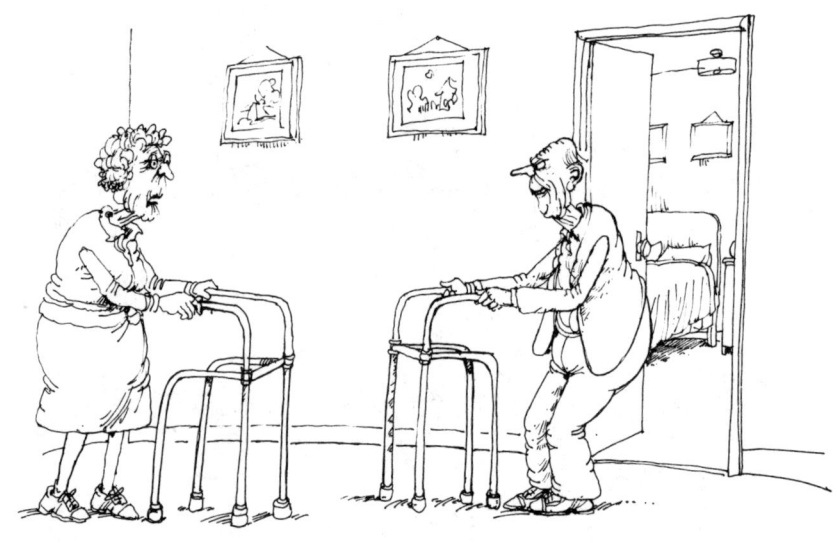

All right — but I'm not doing it standing up.

Some people are stimulated by pornographic magazines . . .

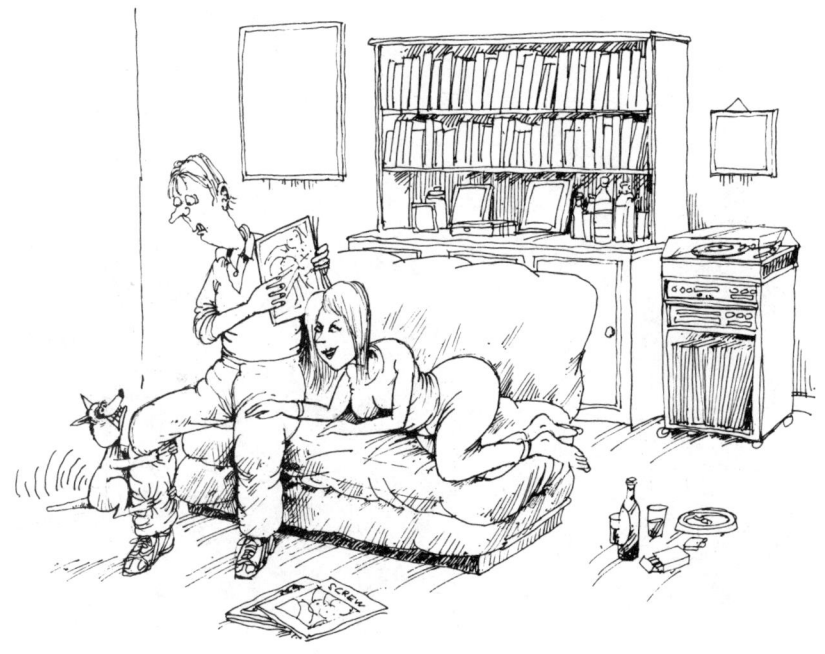

He wants to look at the one with the Alsatian again.

or films.

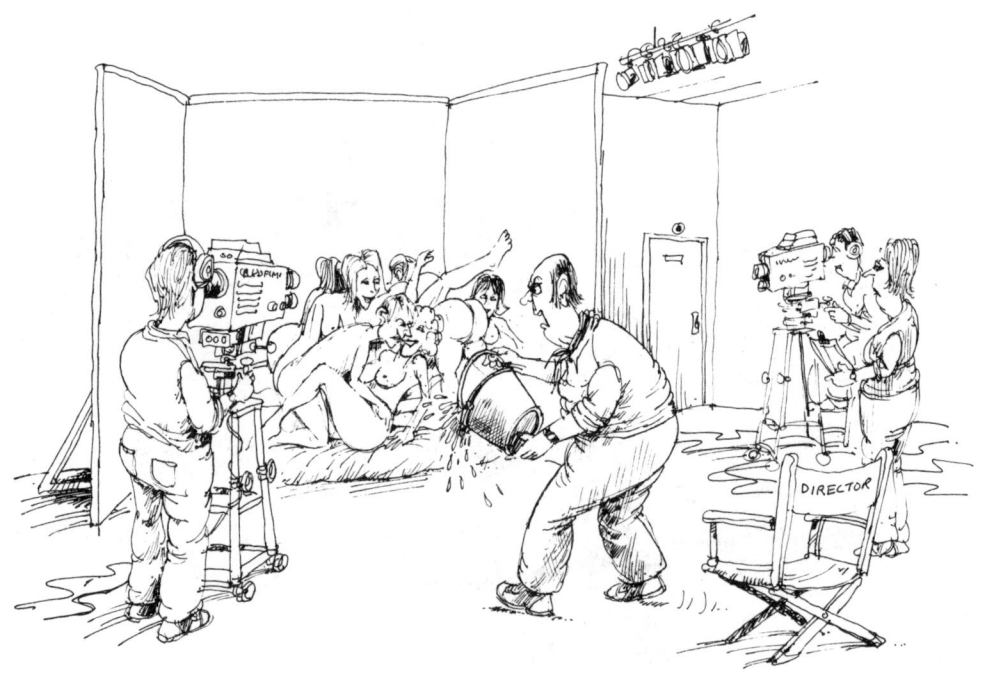

Cut!

Others get their thrills from bondage . . .

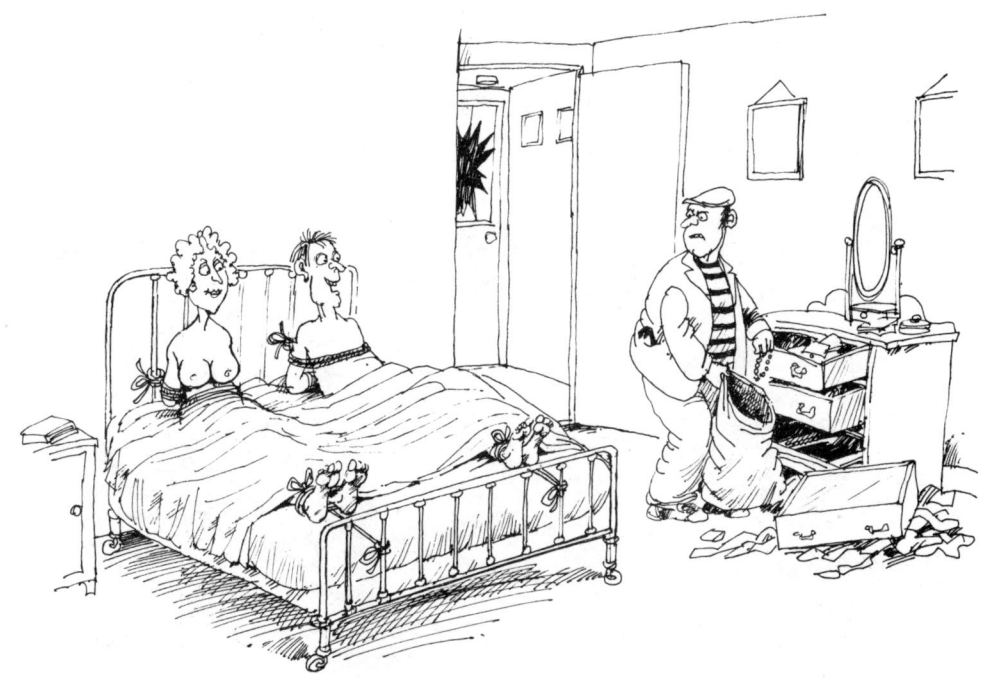

Promise you'll come again.

and flagellation,

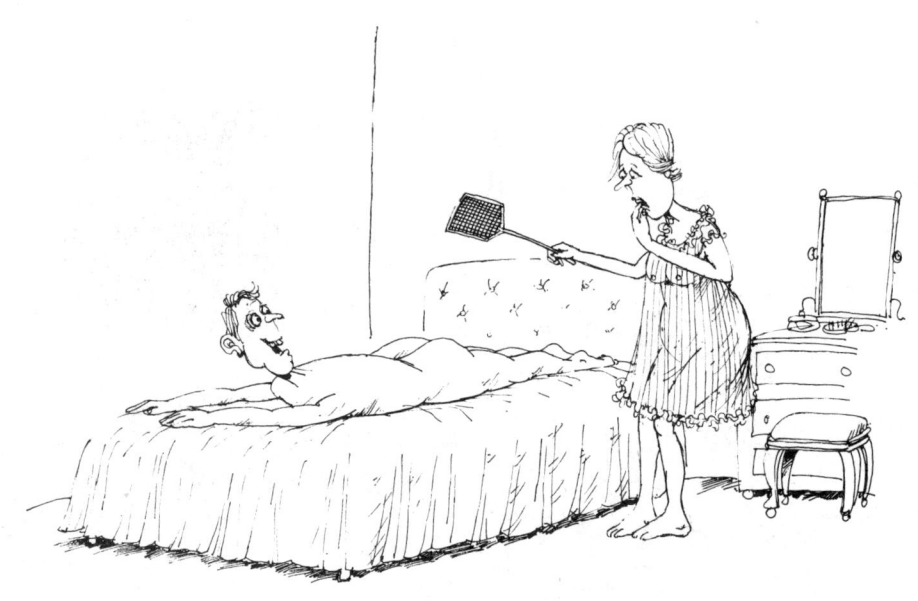

Go on, Mildred — just pretend there's a fly there.

often combined with a fetish for leather or rubber.

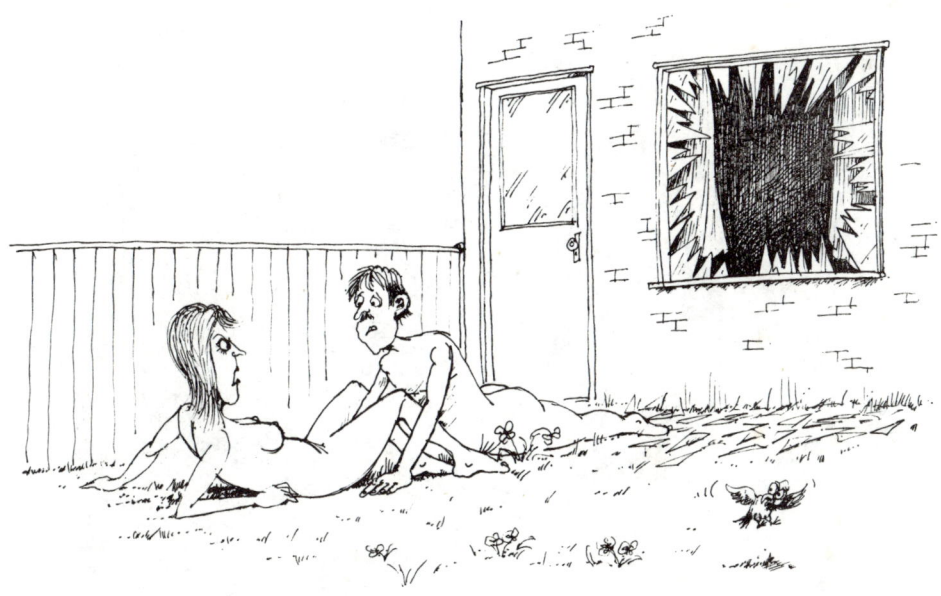

You and your bloody rubber mattress.

There are books and magazines,

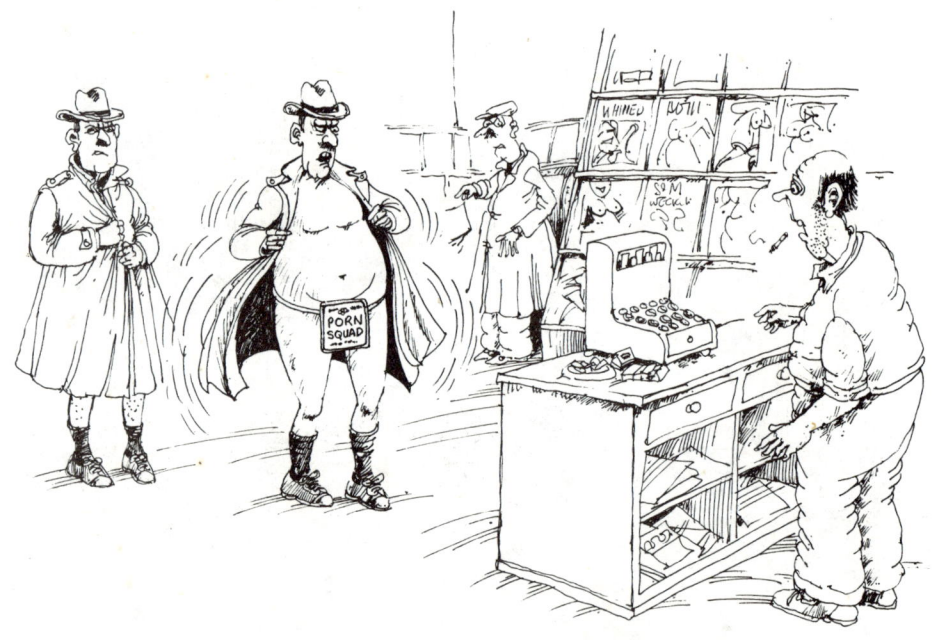

Police — this is a raid!

shops and clubs,

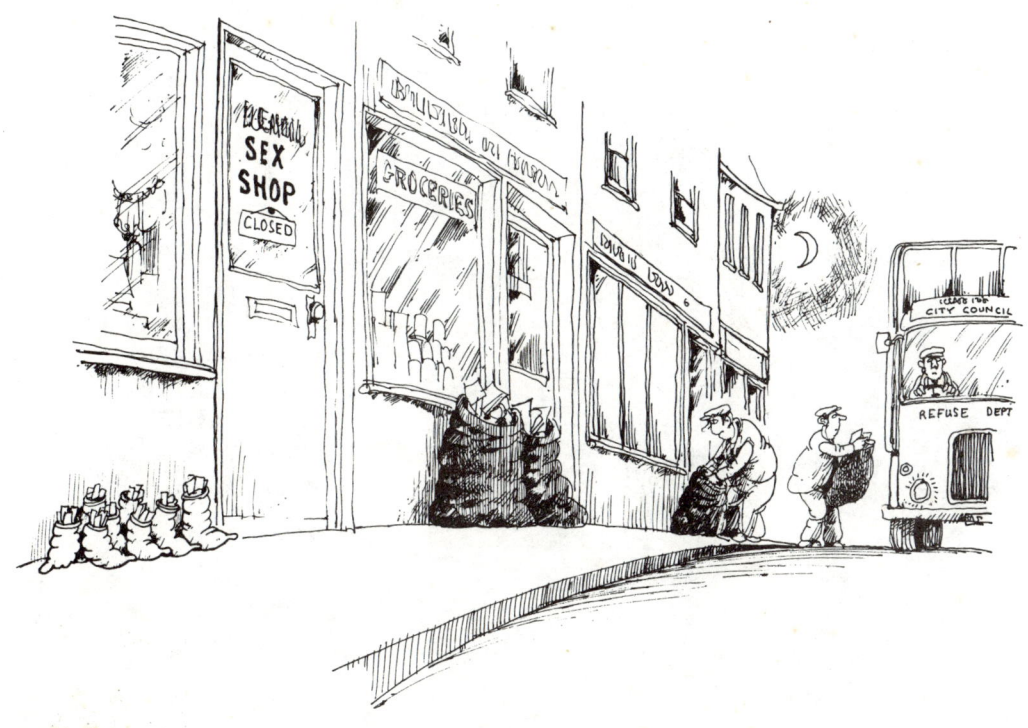

to cater for all tastes.

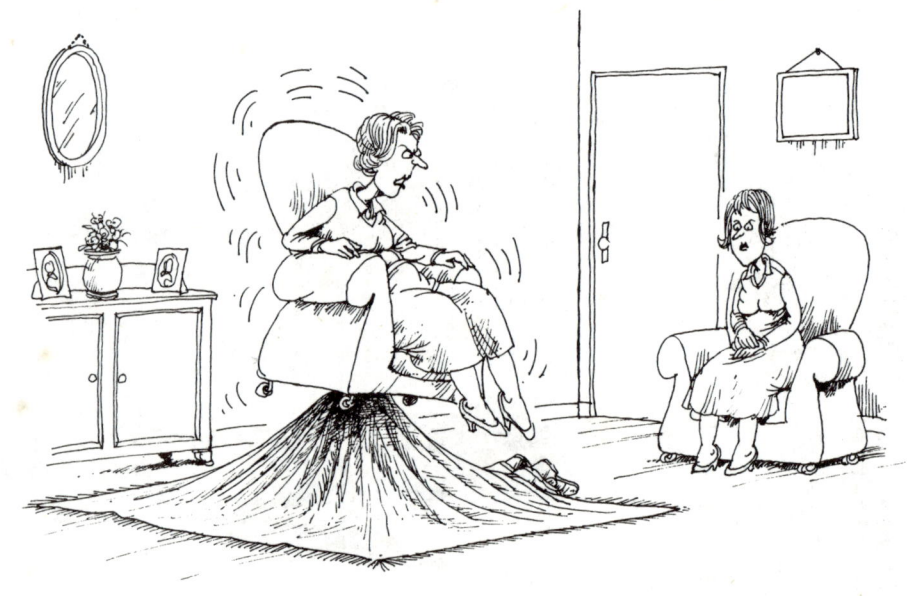

I just wish he'd hide his dirty magazines somewhere else.

However, even in these days of sexual liberation,

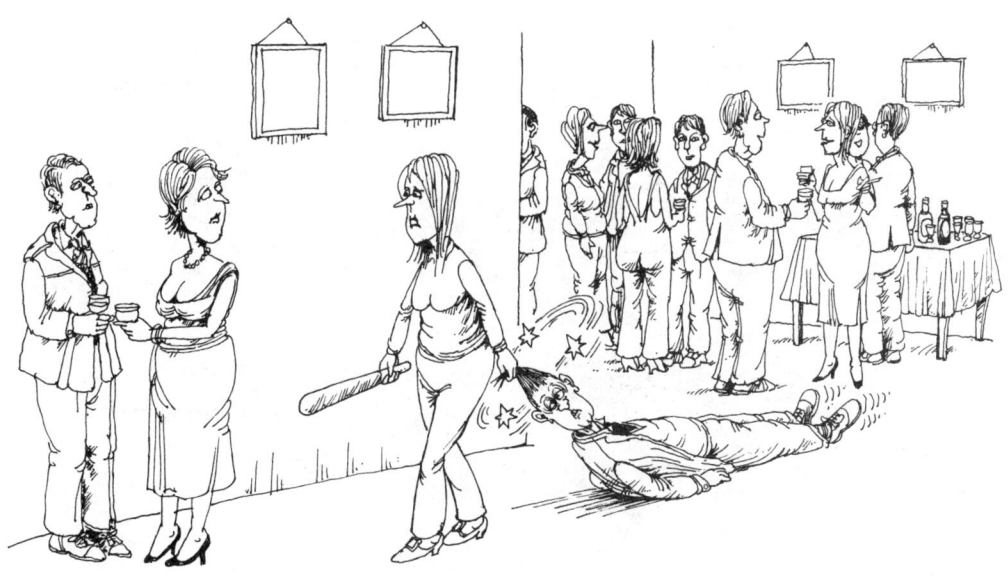

Where's the bedroom?

courtship can still be important . . .

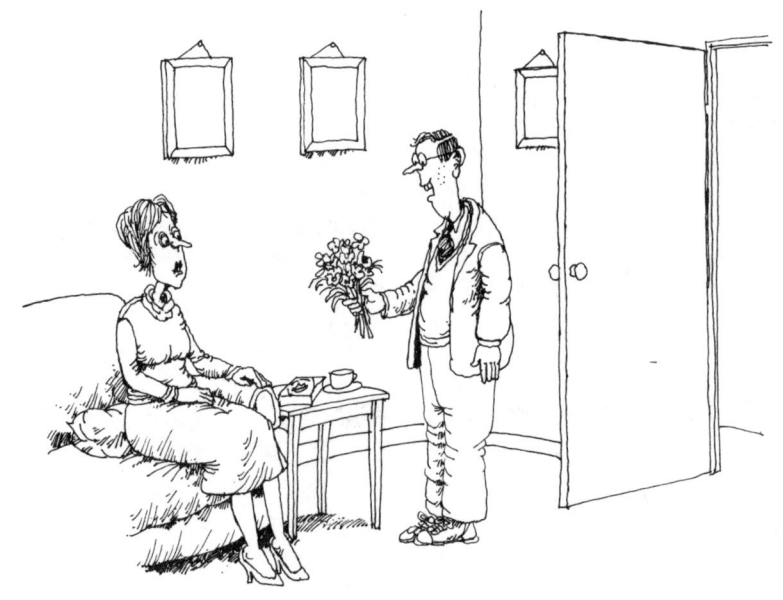

So that our love will last forever, Alice, I've bought you plastic flowers.

— **while some women will happily jump straight into bed,**

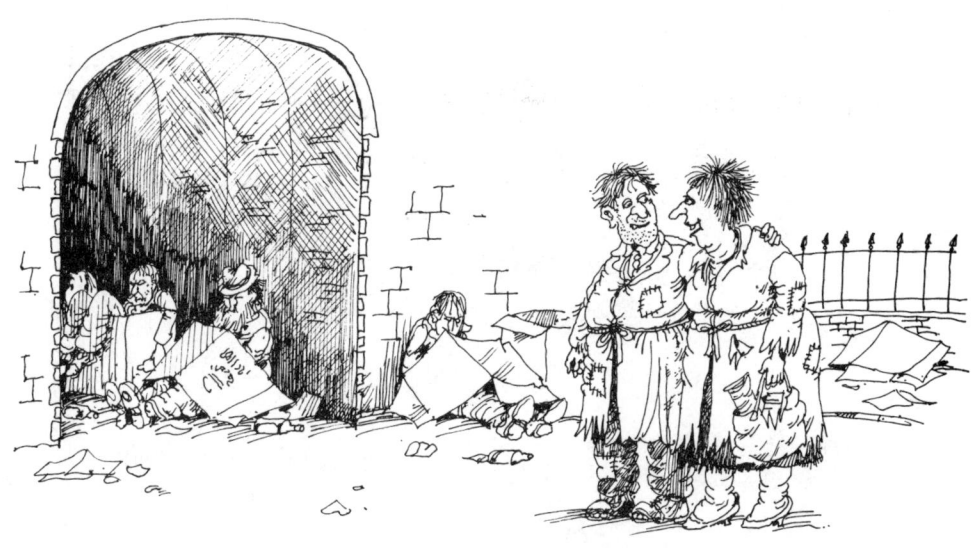

Your box or mine?

others like to be wooed first.

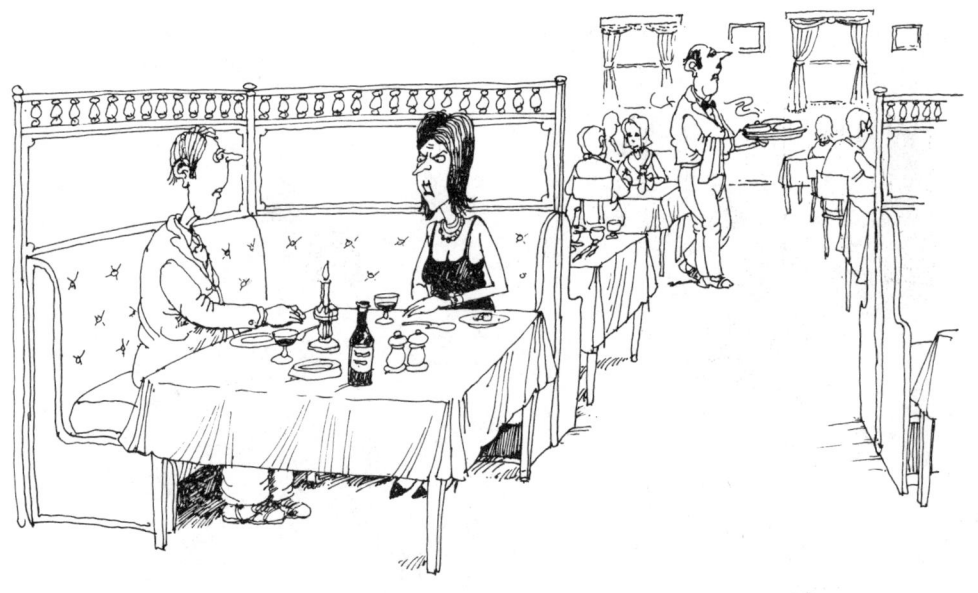

No, I will not have sex with you — at least, not until we've had the dessert.

In some countries there are still strict moral codes . . .

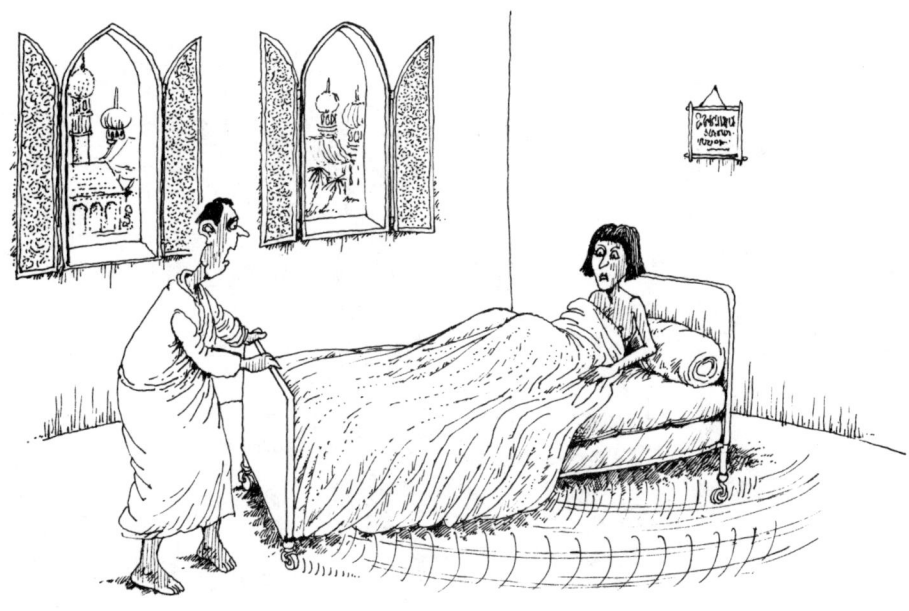

I've just realised we're not facing Mecca.

regarding sexual behaviour,

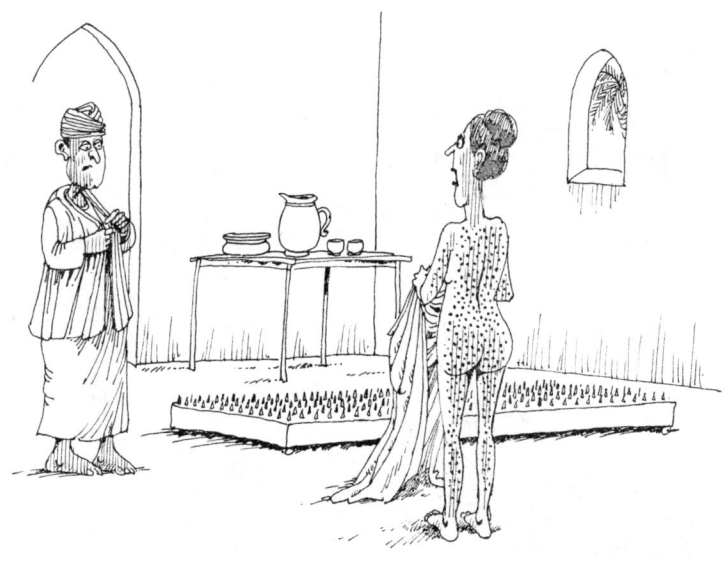

Couldn't I go on top for a change?

and courtship is a ritual . . .

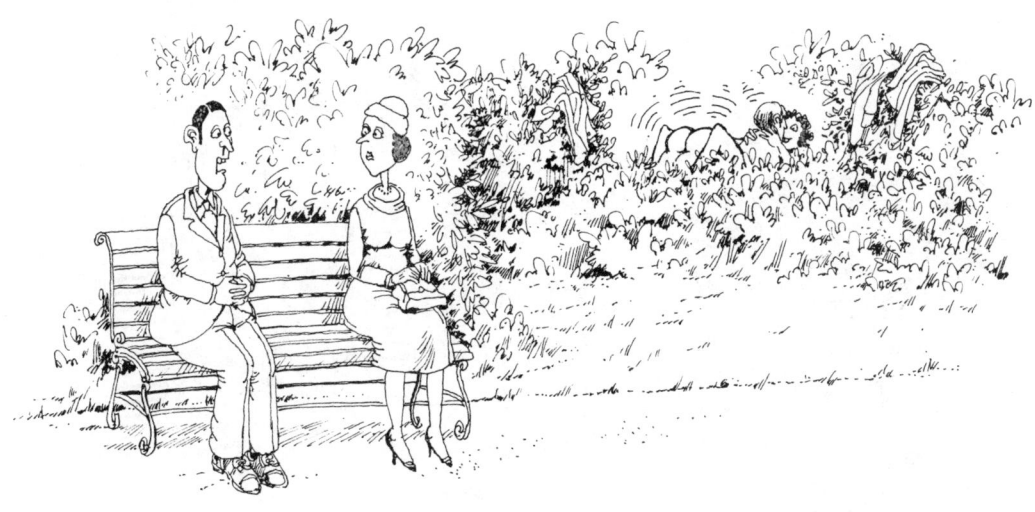

I wonder where our chaperones have got to?

that has to take place over a number of years.

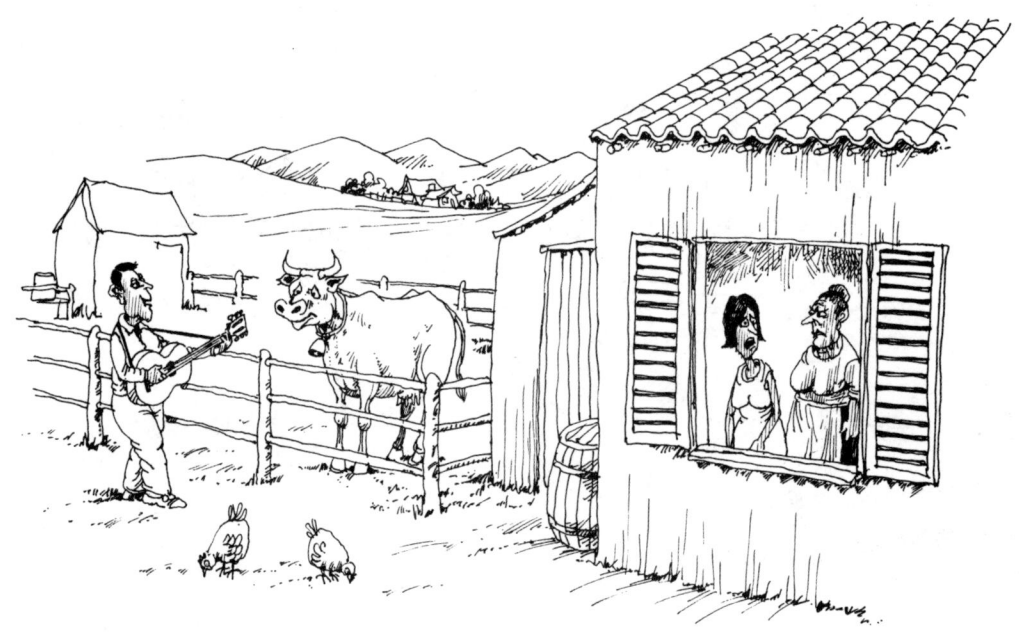

I sometimes think he's more interested in my dowry than in me.

Here, it's more casual . . .

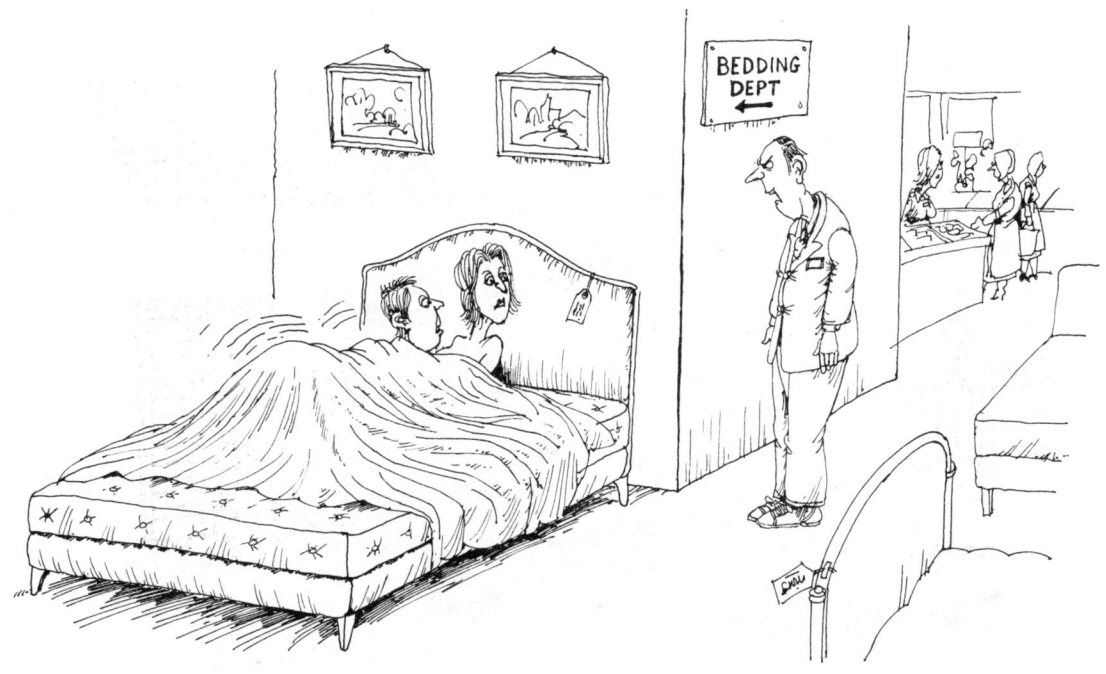

I'm going to transfer you to another department, Miss Brown.

— **though it can still take time.**

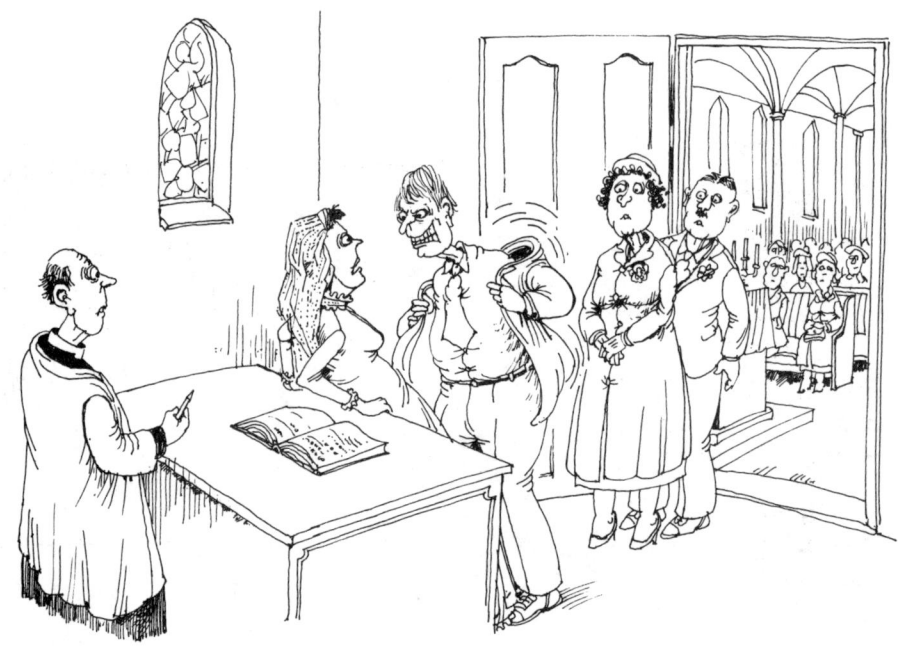

We've waited three years, Harry — a couple more hours won't hurt.

It's not always easy to find the ideal partner . . .

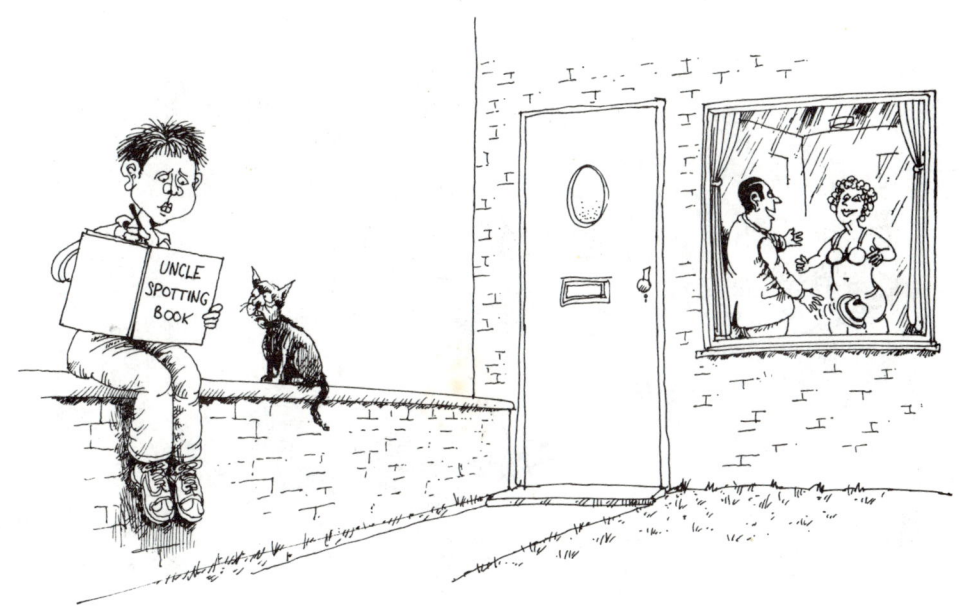

and some never do . . .

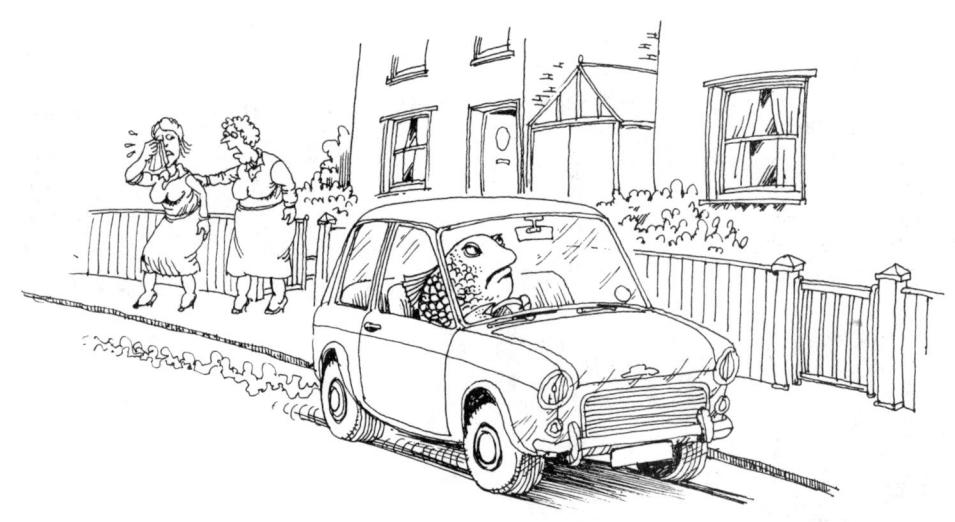

Don't worry, dear, there are plenty of other fish in the sea.

— **but if the usual methods fail . . .**

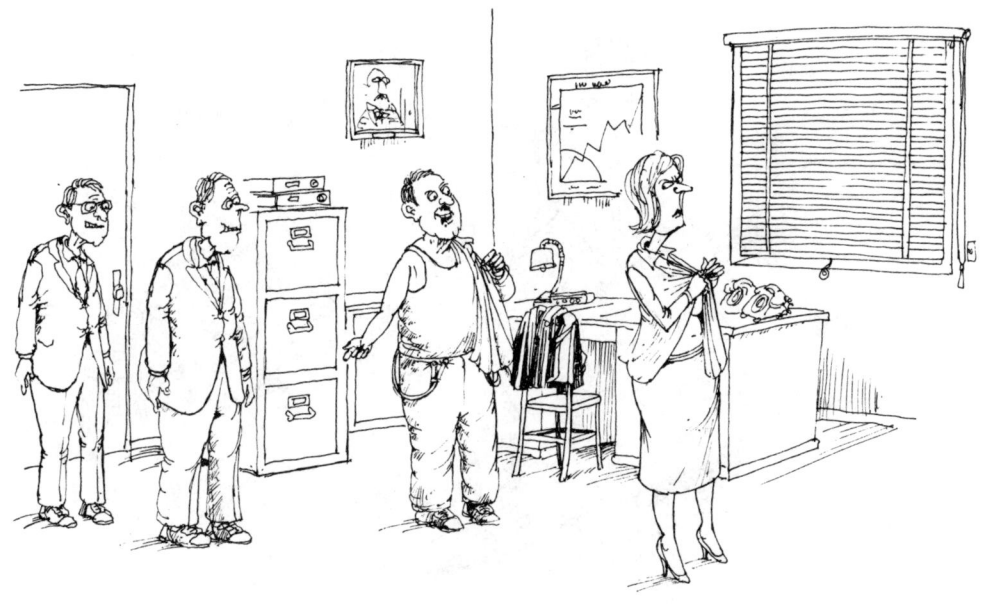

Come on, Miss King — you know everything in this office has to be done in triplicate.

there are dating agencies to help,

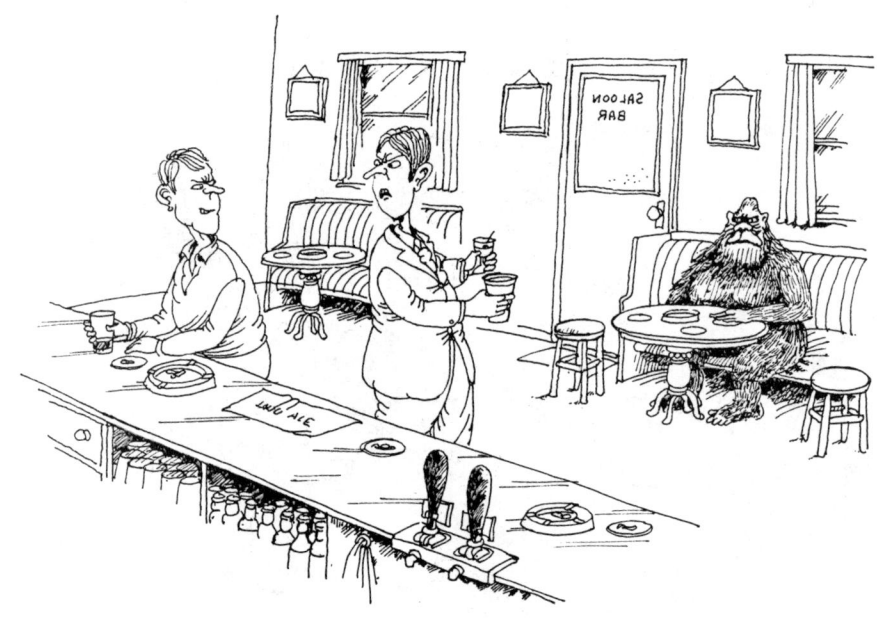

It's the last time I use a computer dating agency.

or you can place advertisements in magazines.

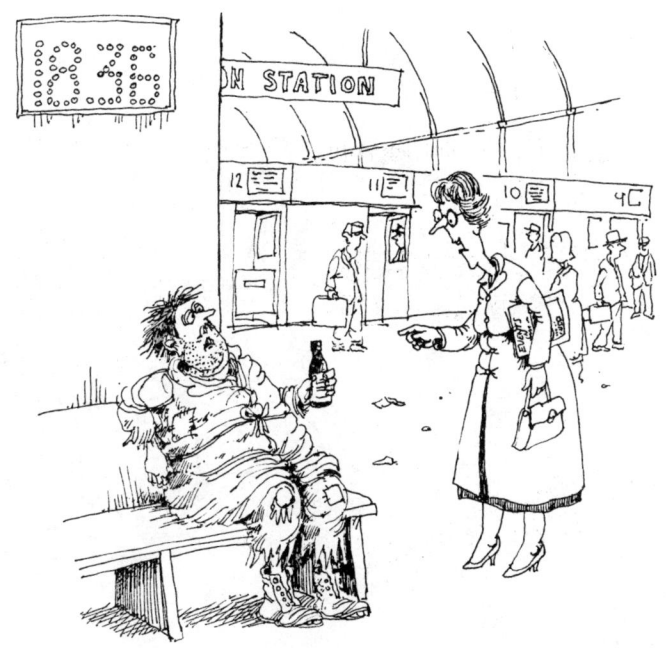

Excuse me, but would you by any chance be 'fun-loving bachelor, enjoys dining out and long walks in the countryside'?

Nowadays it's quite common for couples to live together . . .

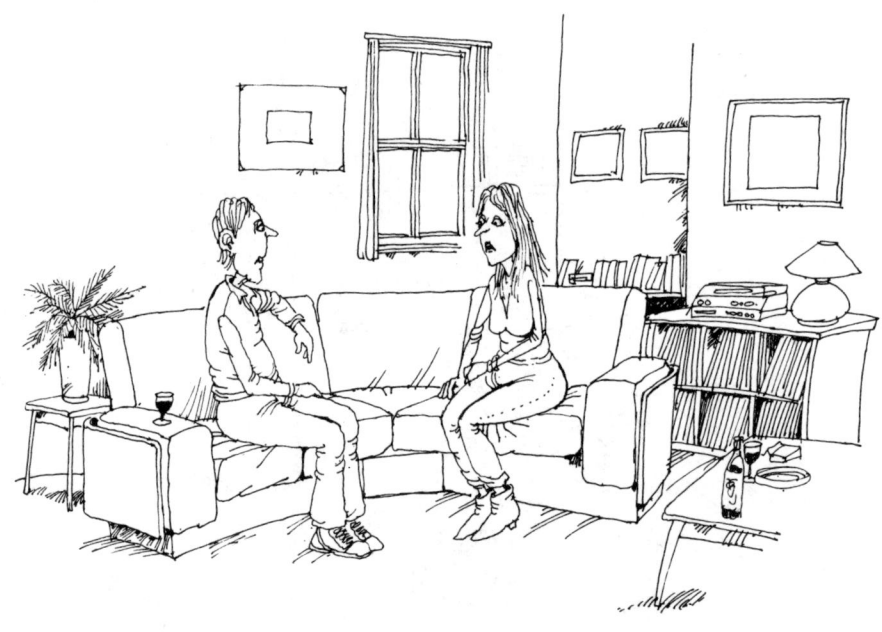

No, I never move in on my first date.

before marriage . . .

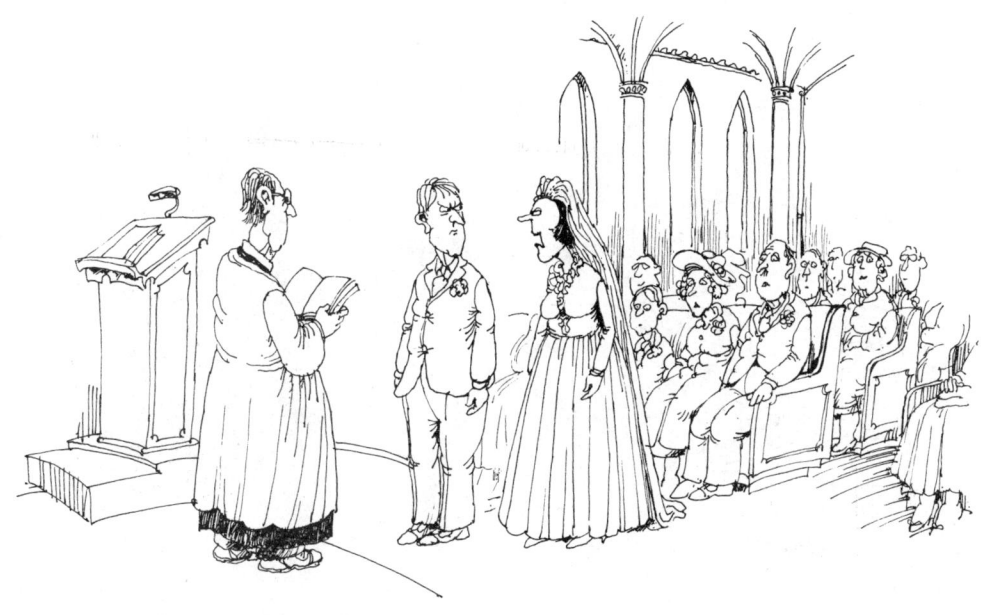

And you left the top off the toothpaste again this morning.

— **or perhaps instead of it.**

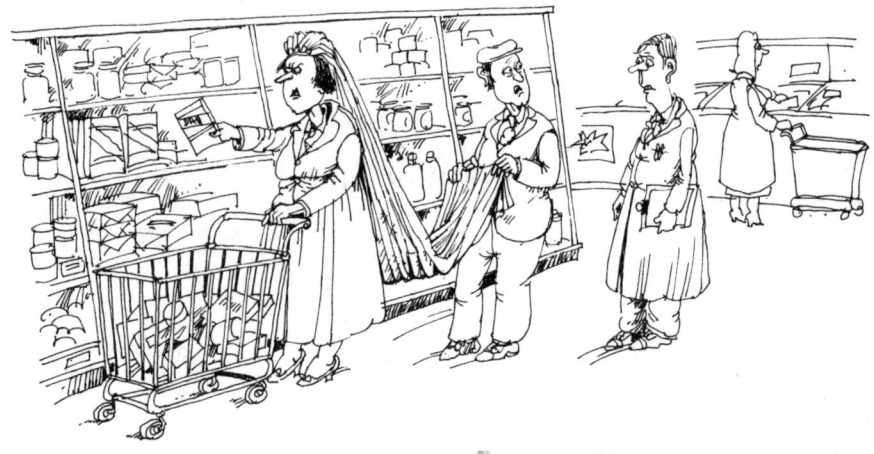

She's going through one of her 'wishing we'd actually got married' phases at the moment.

It's regarded as sensible to be sexually experienced before marriage . . .

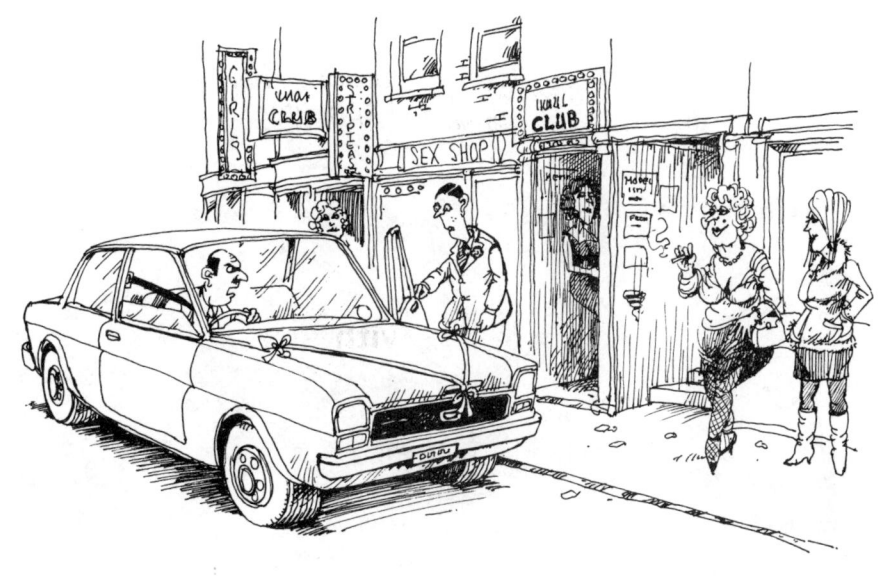

And hurry up — we're supposed to be at the church in five minutes.

and not many brides reach the altar as virgins these days.

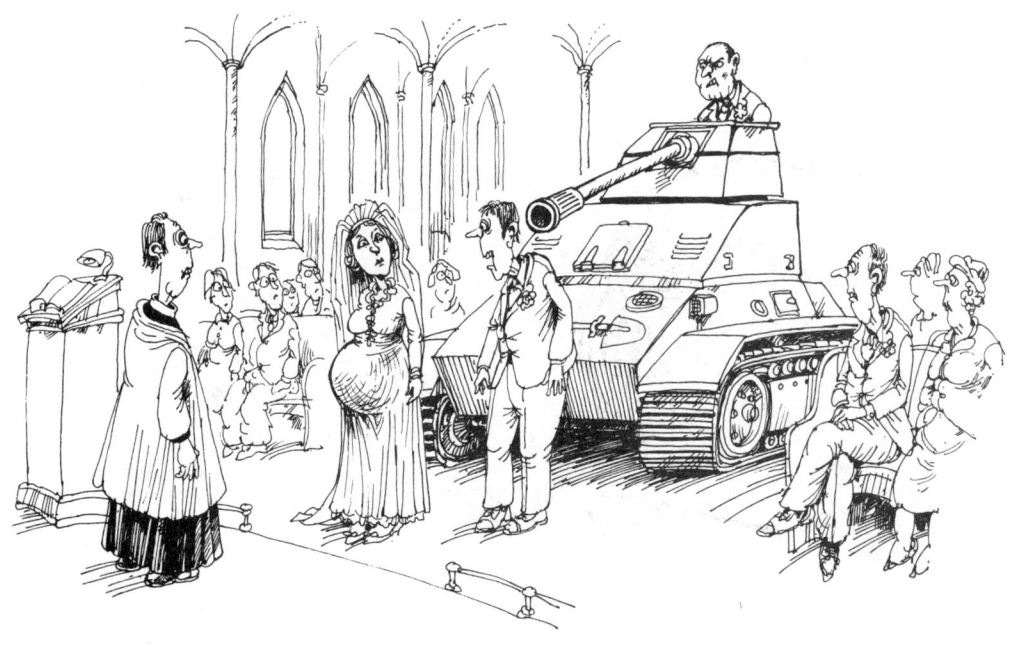

Isn't your father being a little over-dramatic?

Of course, sex is equally important after marriage . . .

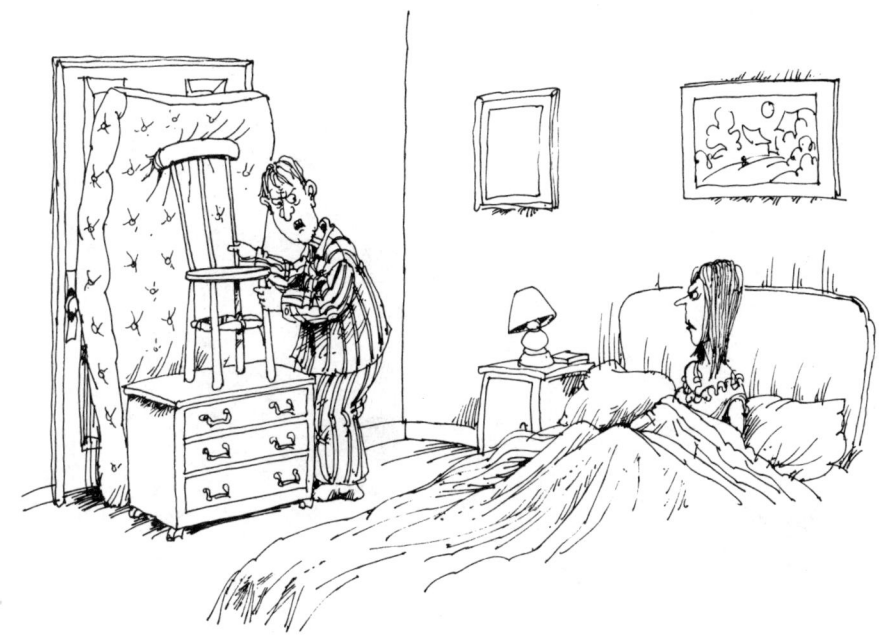

Is this really necessary? I'm sure the children are fast asleep.

— **but it often gets taken for granted . . .**

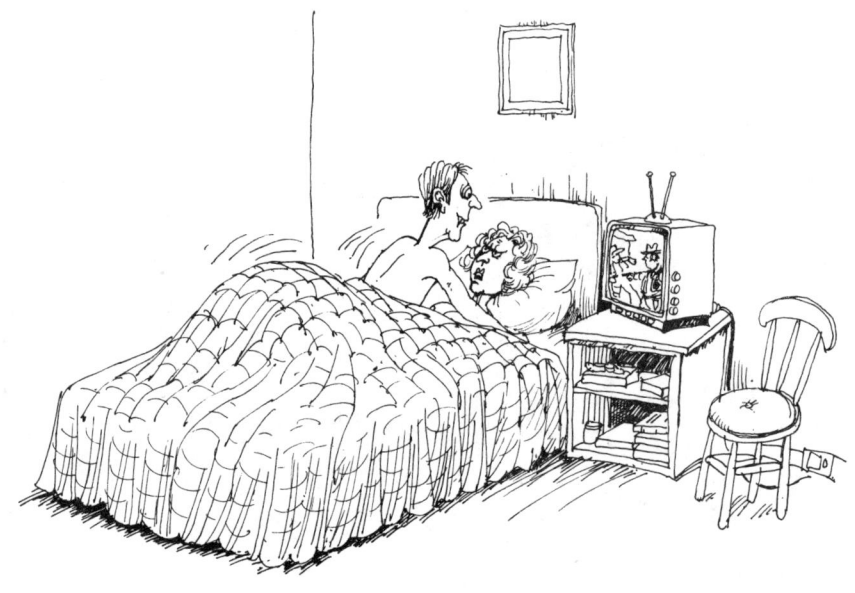

Hasn't it ever occurred to you that I might like to watch television as well?

and after a number of years can become a boring routine.

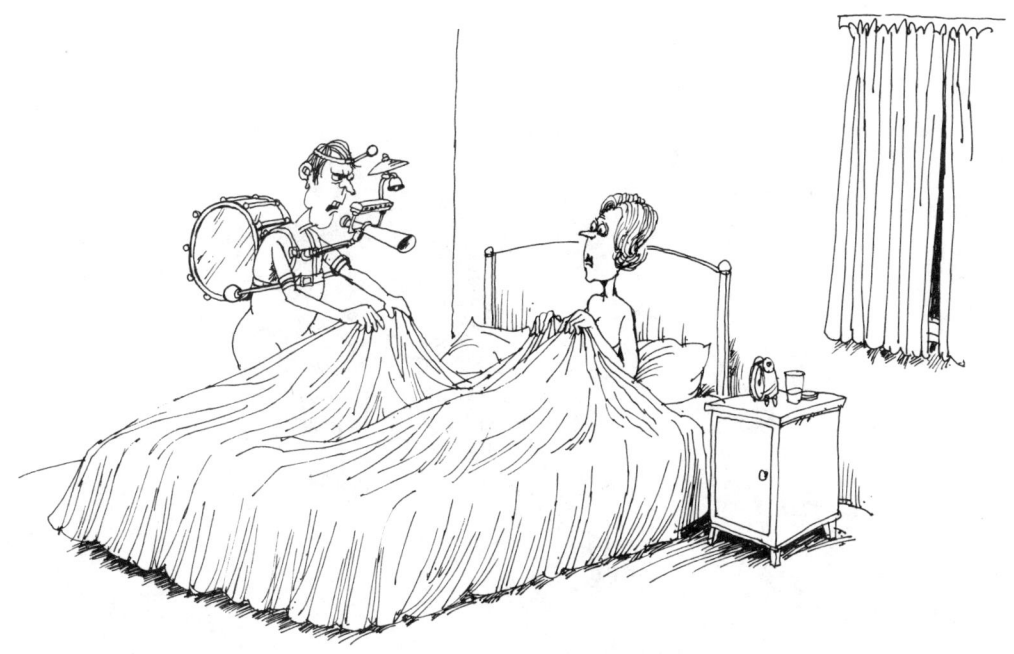

You won't go to sleep on me this time.

Some couples take steps to prevent this . . .

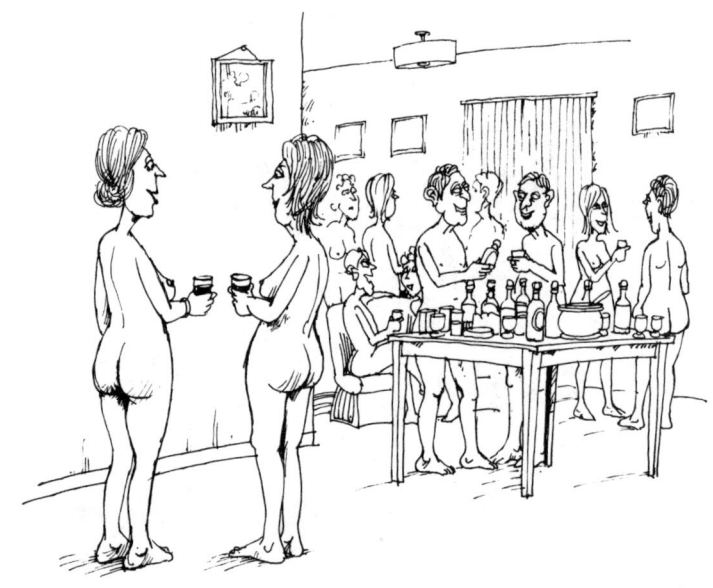

What I love about your parties, Norma, is never having to worry about what to wear.

and to enliven their sex lives.

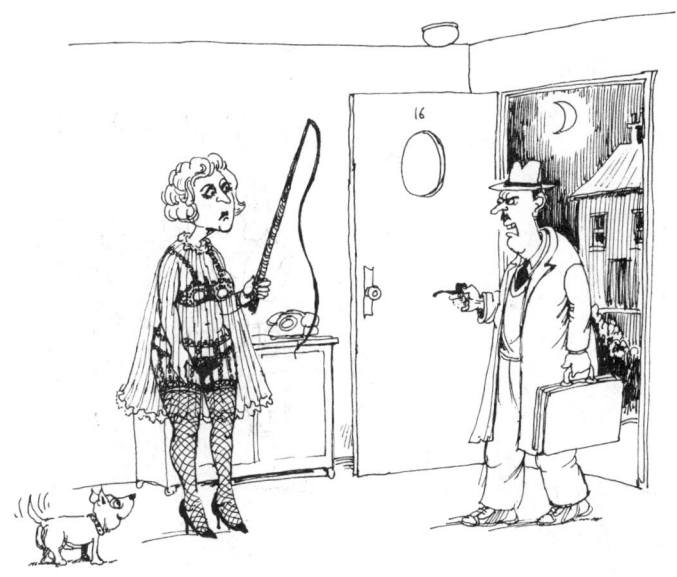

Never mind that — what's for dinner?

They might seek a change of partner . . .

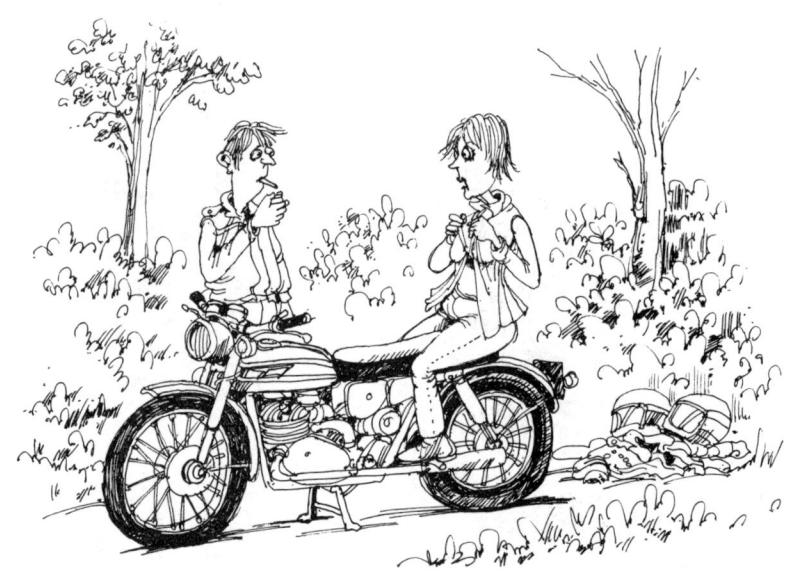

I thought the back seat of Brian's car was bad enough . . .

— **with the other's knowledge,**

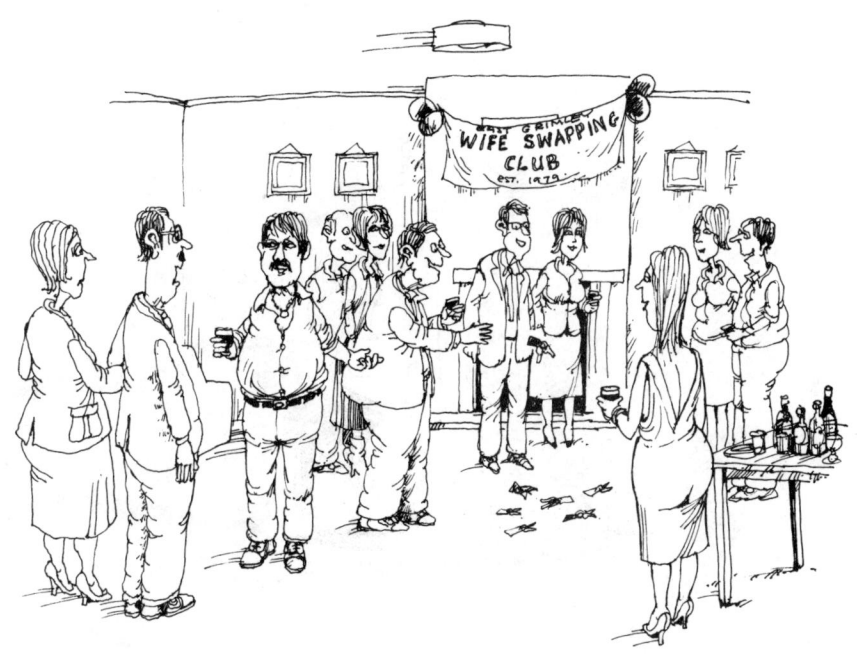

We haven't got a car — is it all right if we throw our bus tickets in the middle?

or without it.

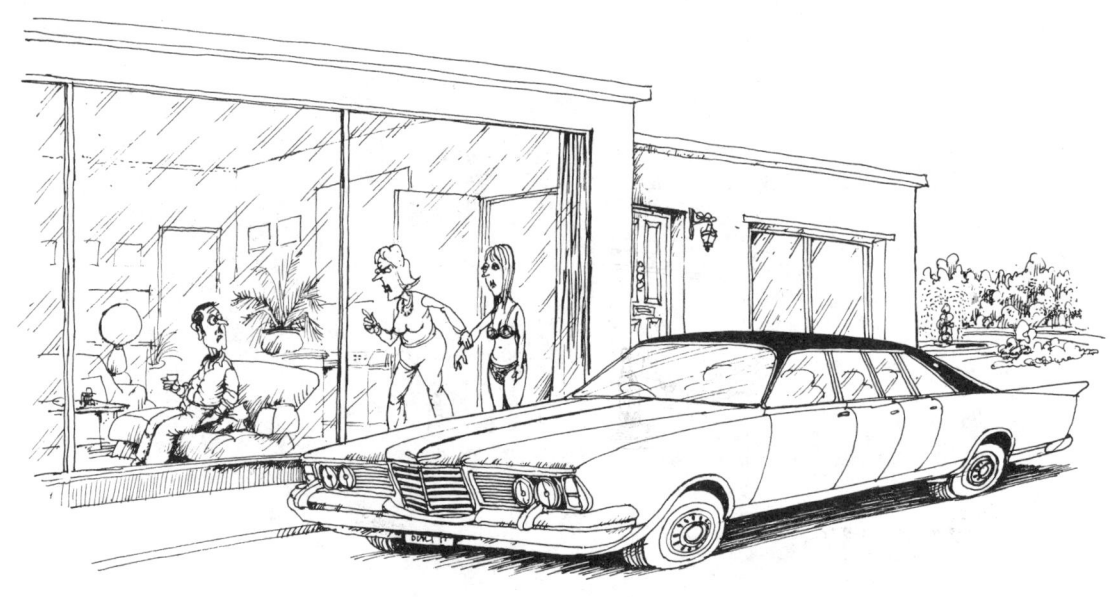

Don't lie to me, Harry — I found this in the glove compartment of the car.

Sometimes this can help a relationship,

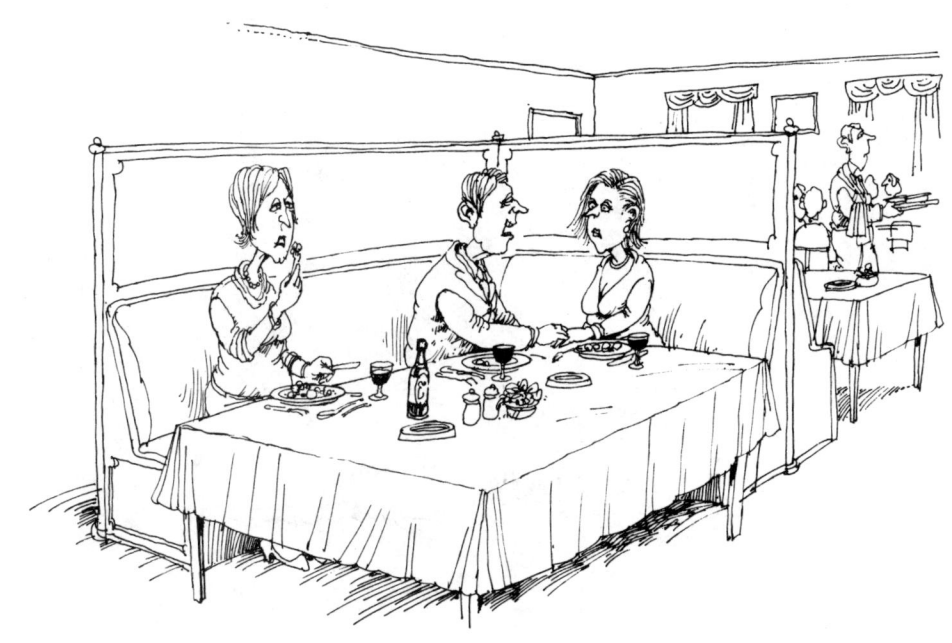

Actually, my wife does understand me.

often it will destroy it.

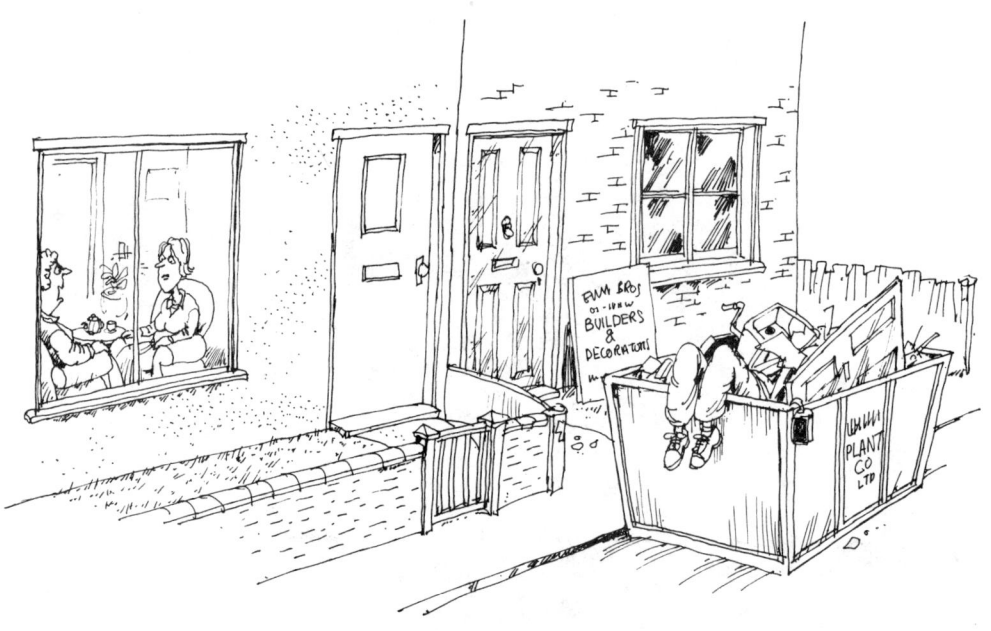

You finally threw him out, then?

Sexual problems are often given . . .

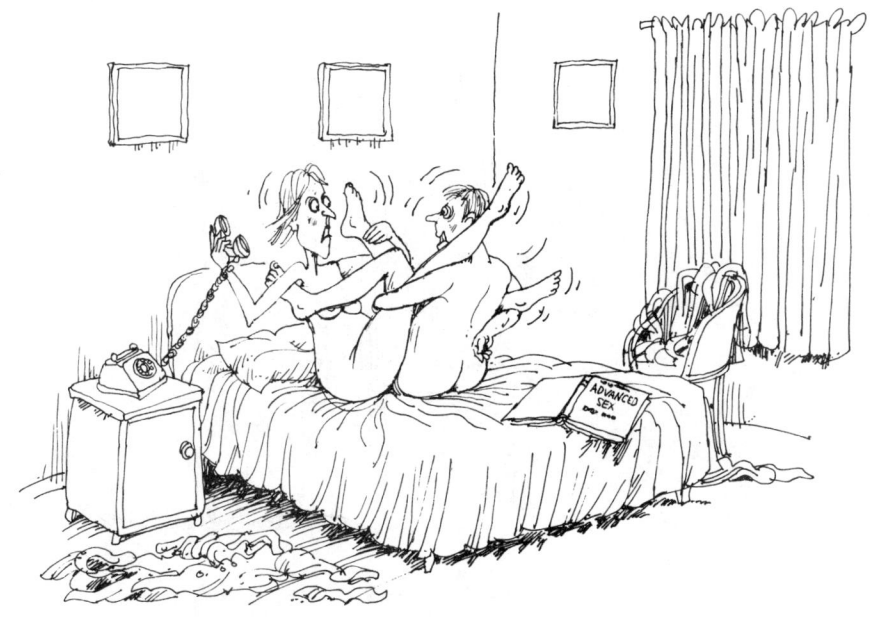

Which service should I ask for?

as the reason for a marriage break-up.

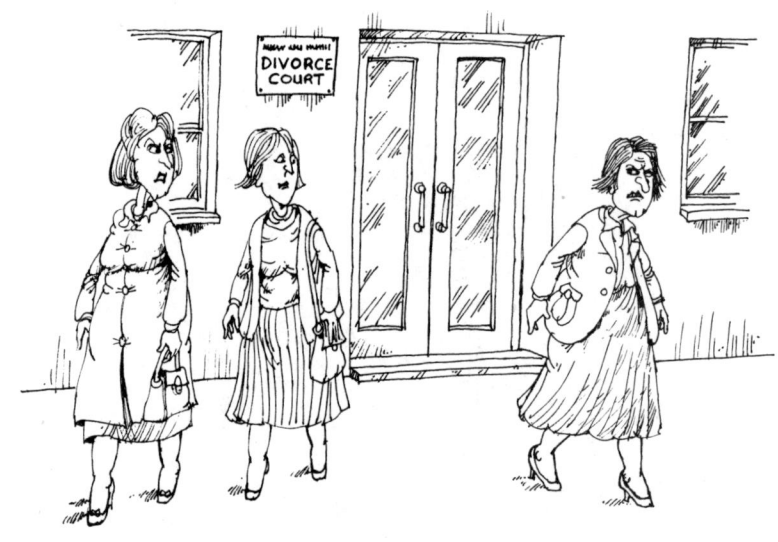

I wouldn't have minded if he'd bought his own clothes instead of wearing mine.

Despite today's sexual freedom,

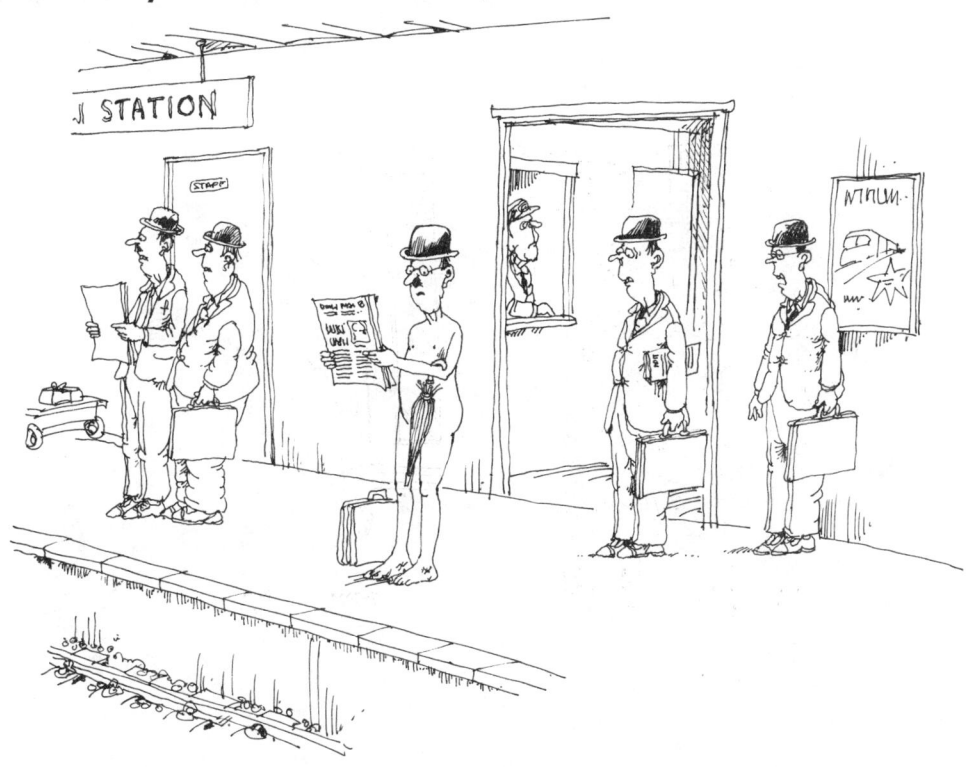

Dobson is terrified the permissive age will pass him by.

many people still have problems with sex,

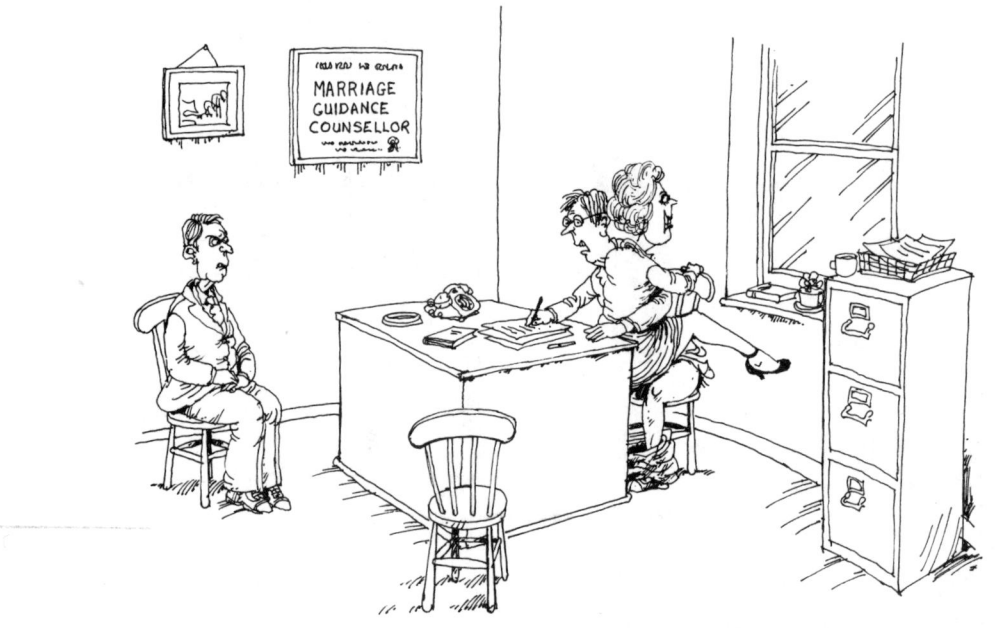

Is there anything else, Mr Dobson, apart from her insatiable sexual appetite?

most of them psychological . . .

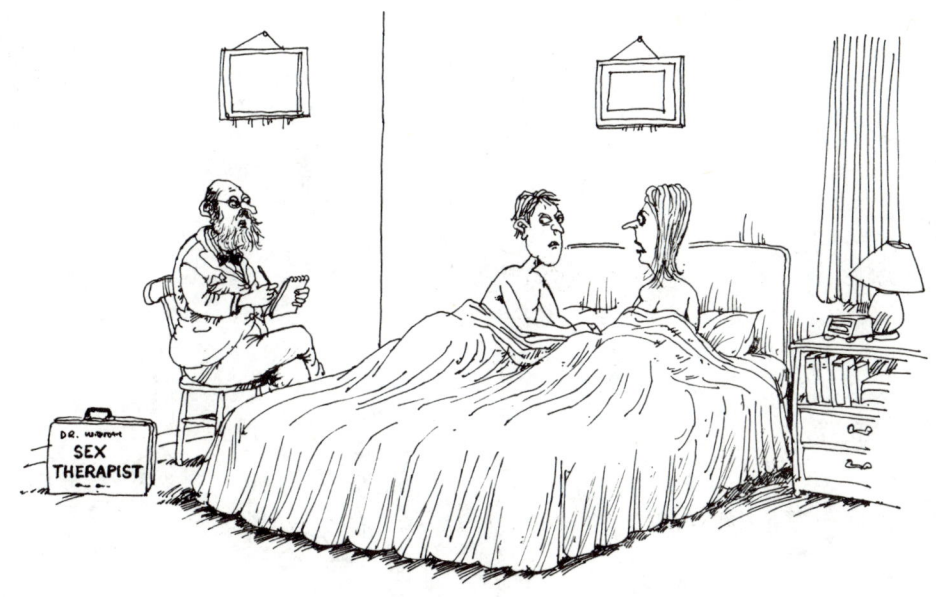

With the amount he charges per hour, it's no wonder you still finish too quickly.

— leading to impotence . . .

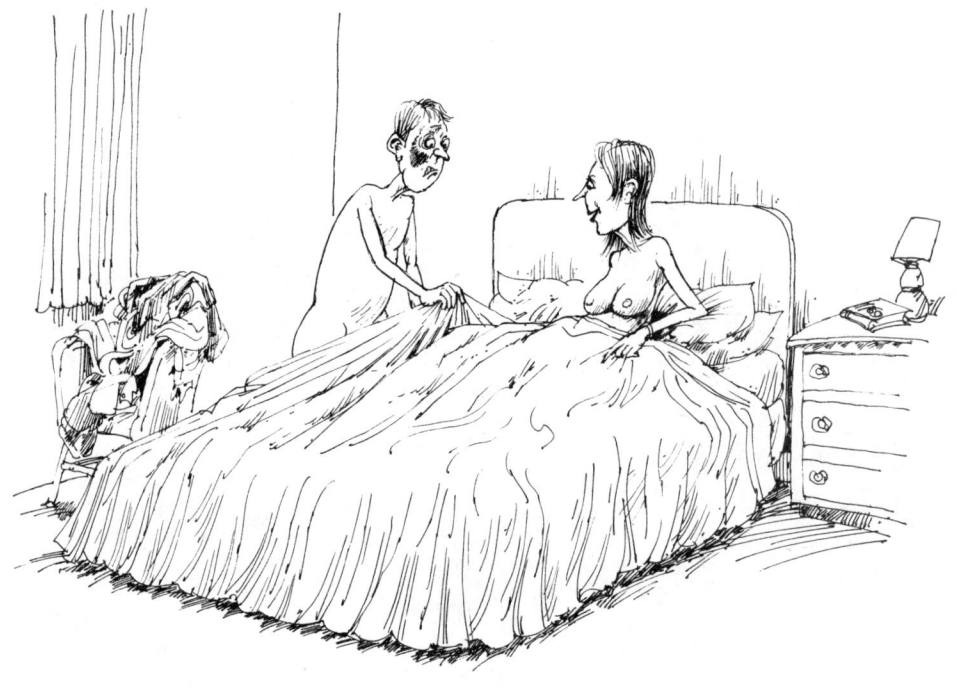

You're not going to let a little thing like that come between us?

or frigidity.

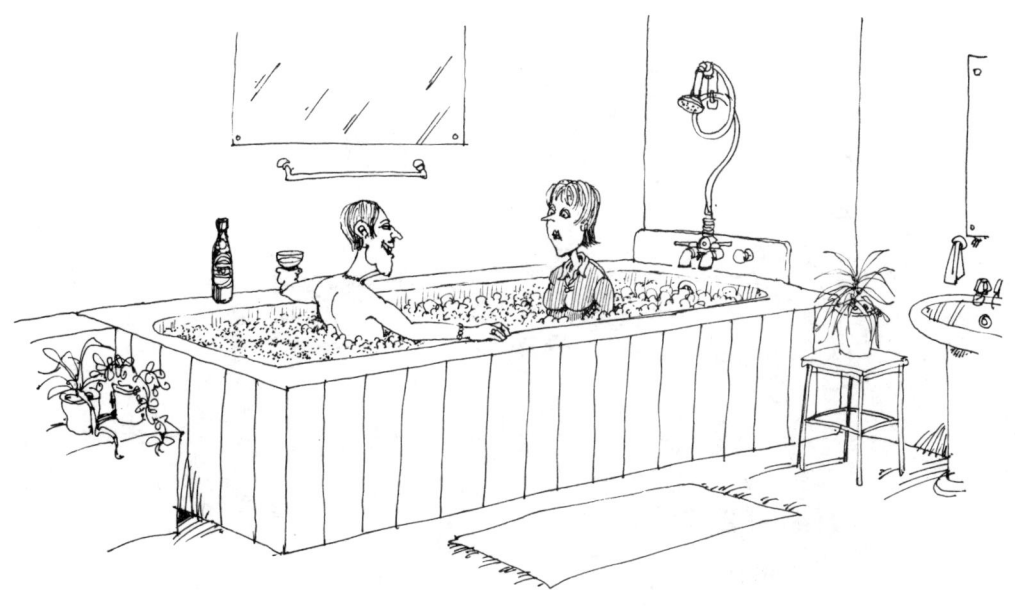

*You must try and rid yourself of these inhibitions,
Violet.*

Help is at hand . . .

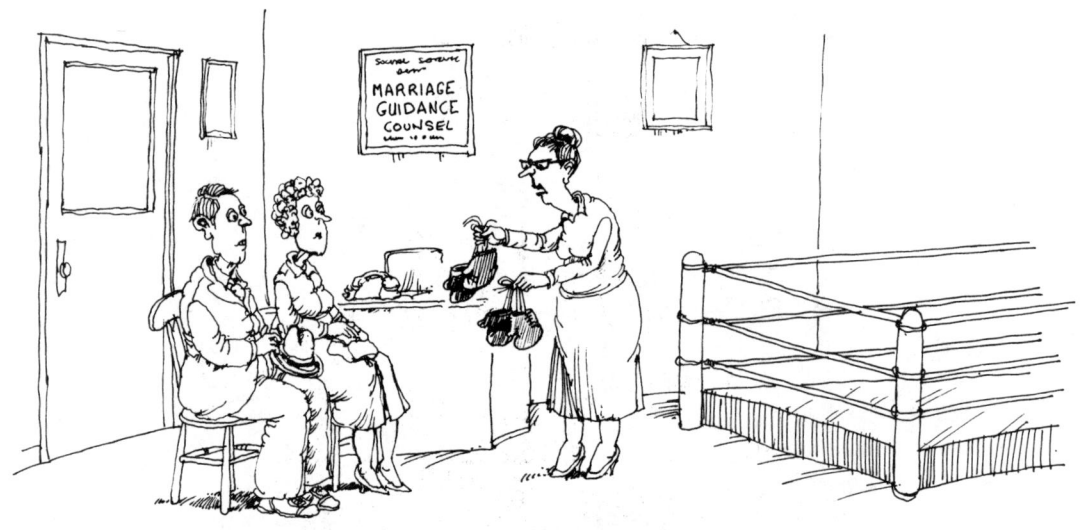

Personally, I don't think talking about it does much good.

for those wishing to seek it.

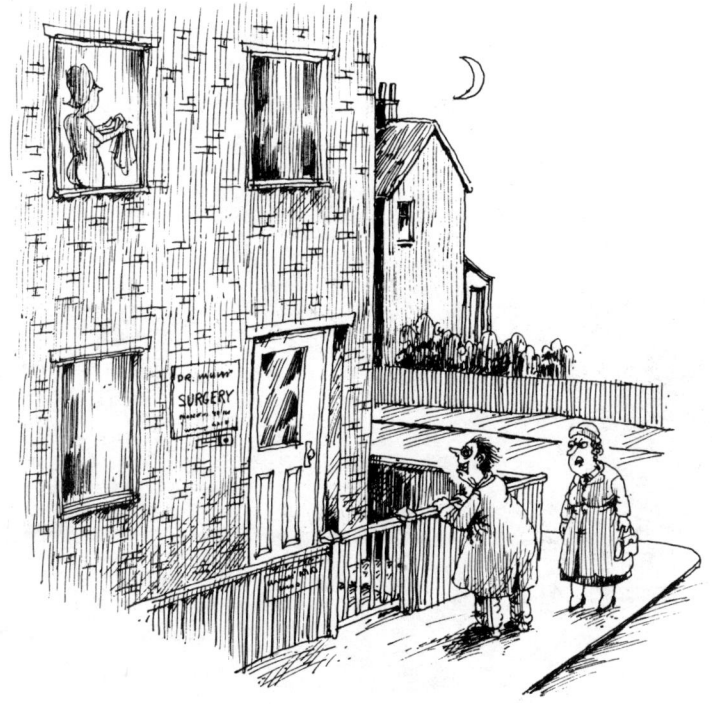

This isn't quite what I meant when I said you ought to see a doctor.

Some sex experts, however, are voicing concern.

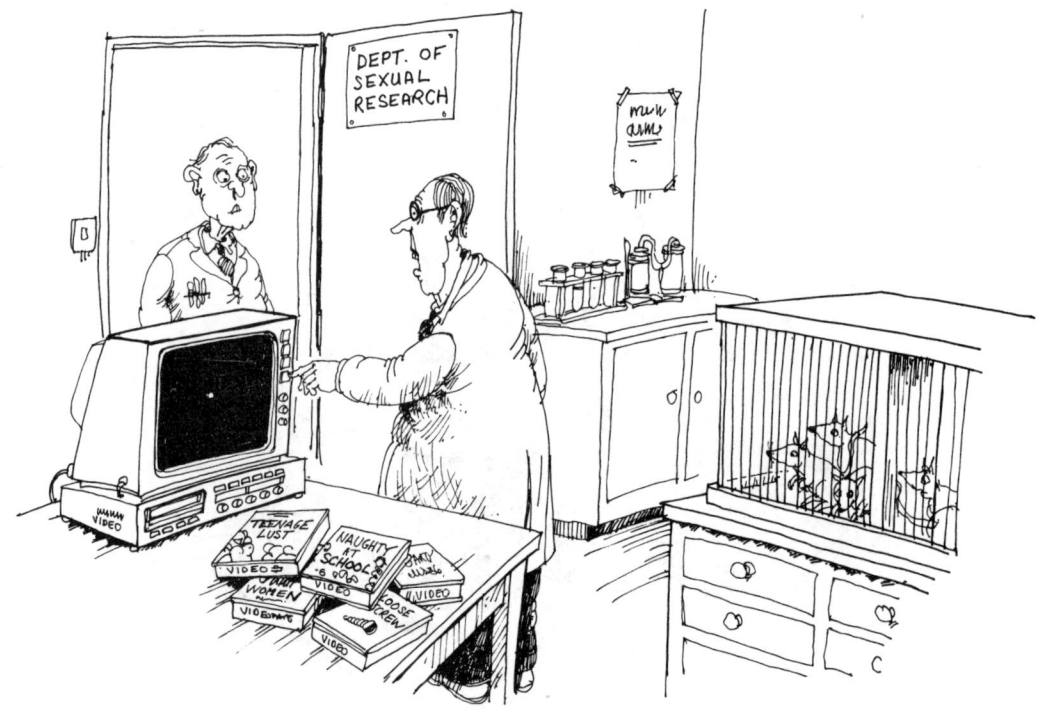

I'm getting worried, Bill — we can't arouse the rats any more.

They worry that the pendulum has swung too far . . .

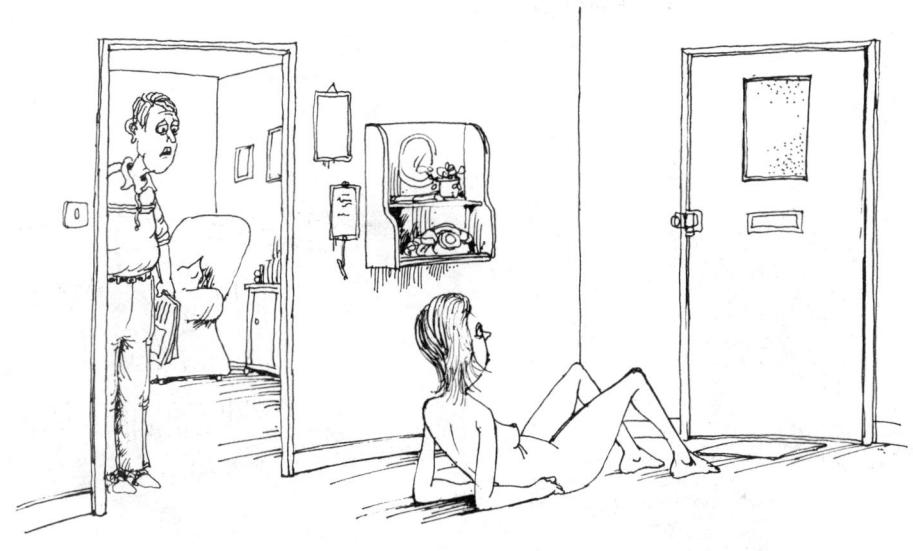

Are you waiting for anyone in particular, dear?

and that sex has been reduced to a mechanical level.

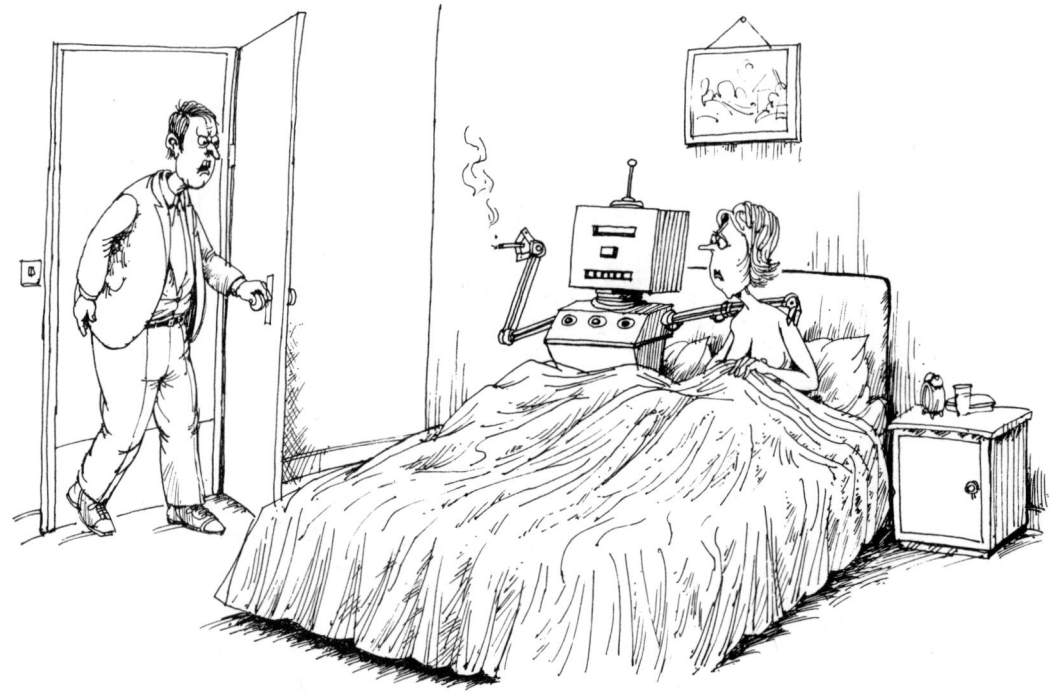

Taking over my job was one thing . . .

Love and feelings, they say, are just as important . . .

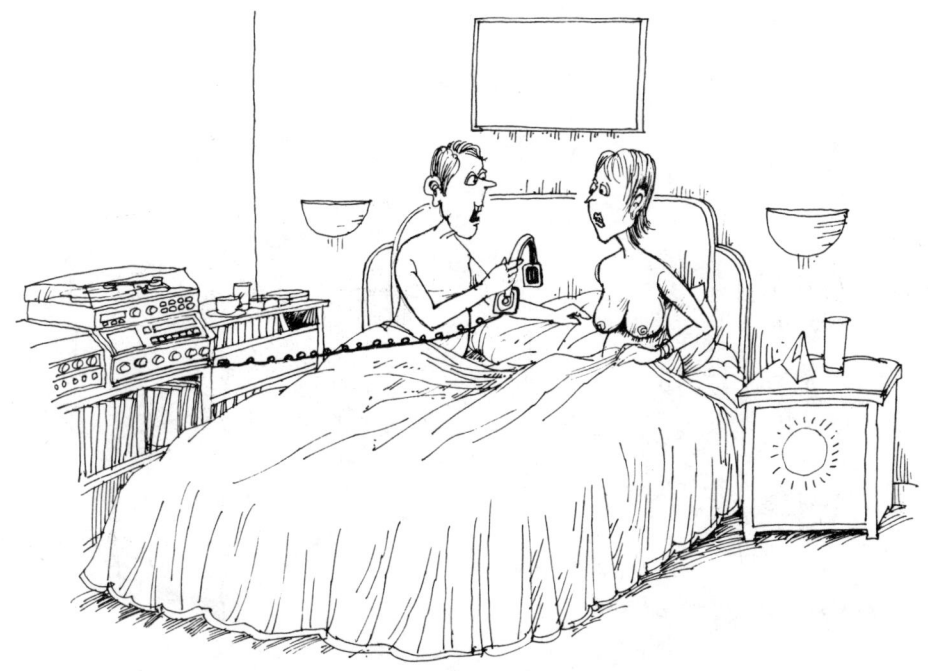

Wear these and I'll put on a tape of sweet nothings.

as sexual gymnastics.

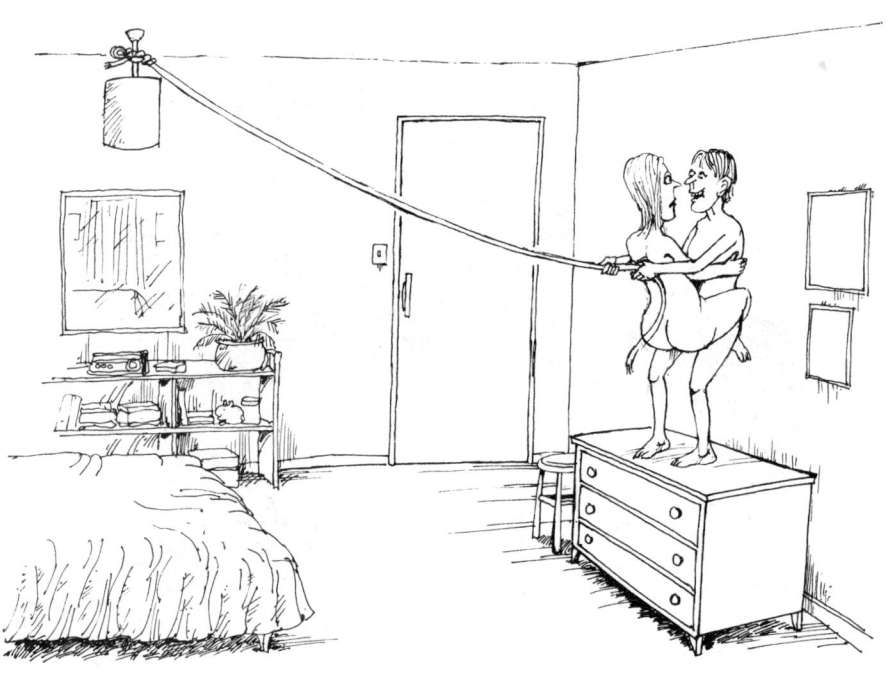

I call this the Tarzan position.

More romance is needed . . .

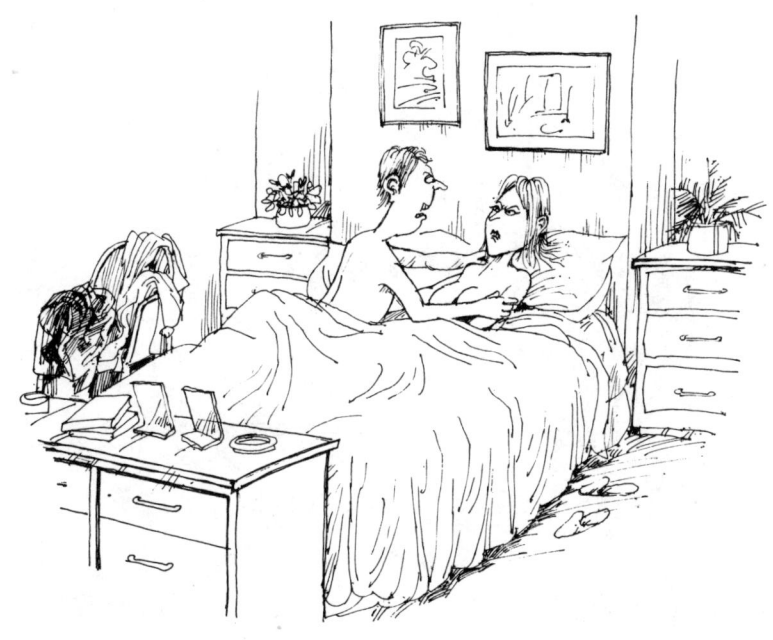

I said 'hello' — what more do you want?

— **and more restraint.**

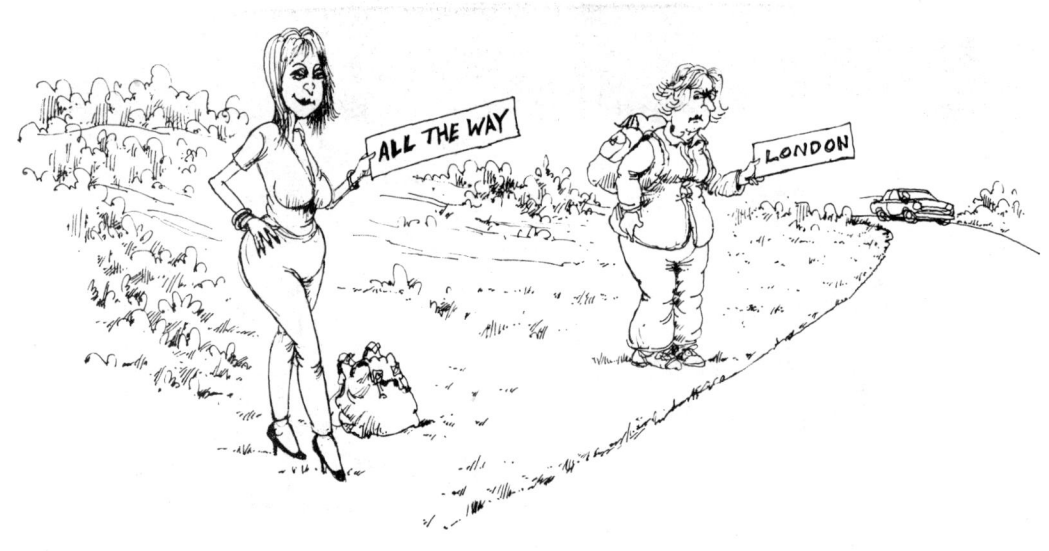

With so much emphasis on sex,

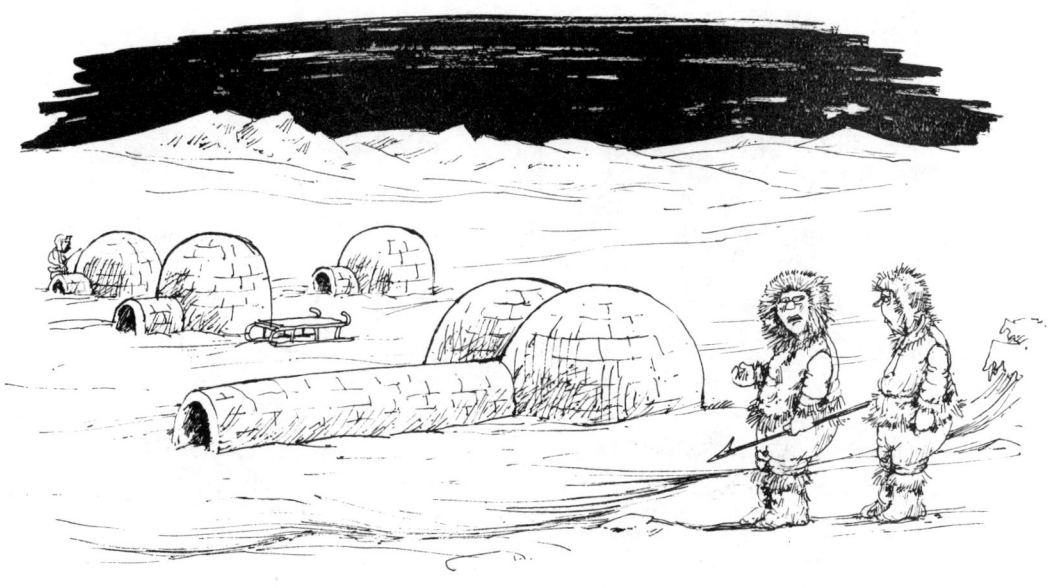

Chinook fancies himself as a bit of a stud.

perhaps people have been taking it too seriously.

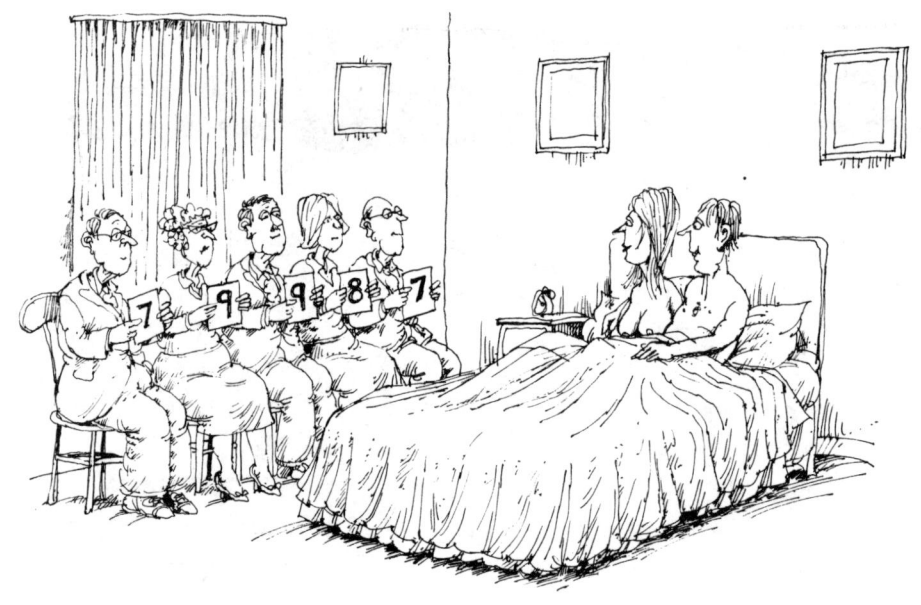

After all, above everything else,

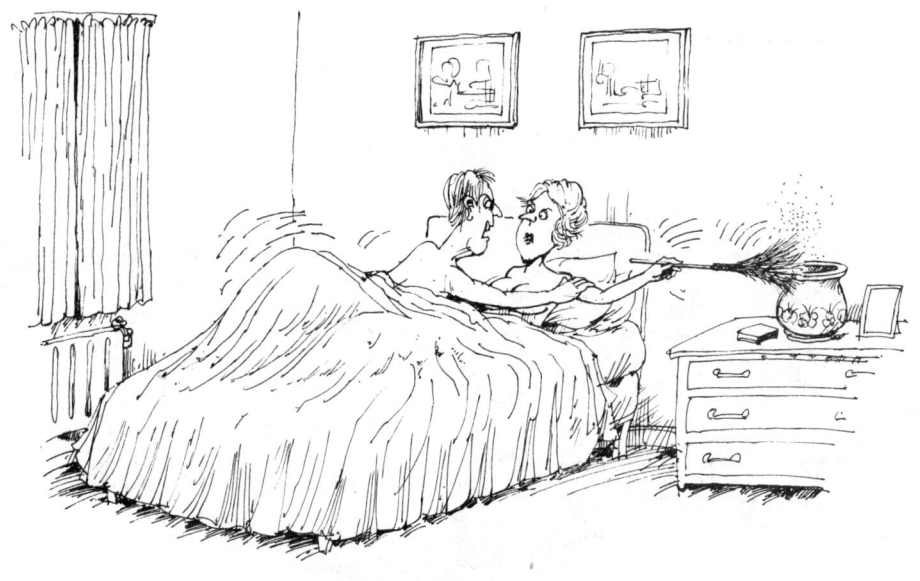

I said 'forget the housework'.

it should be fun.

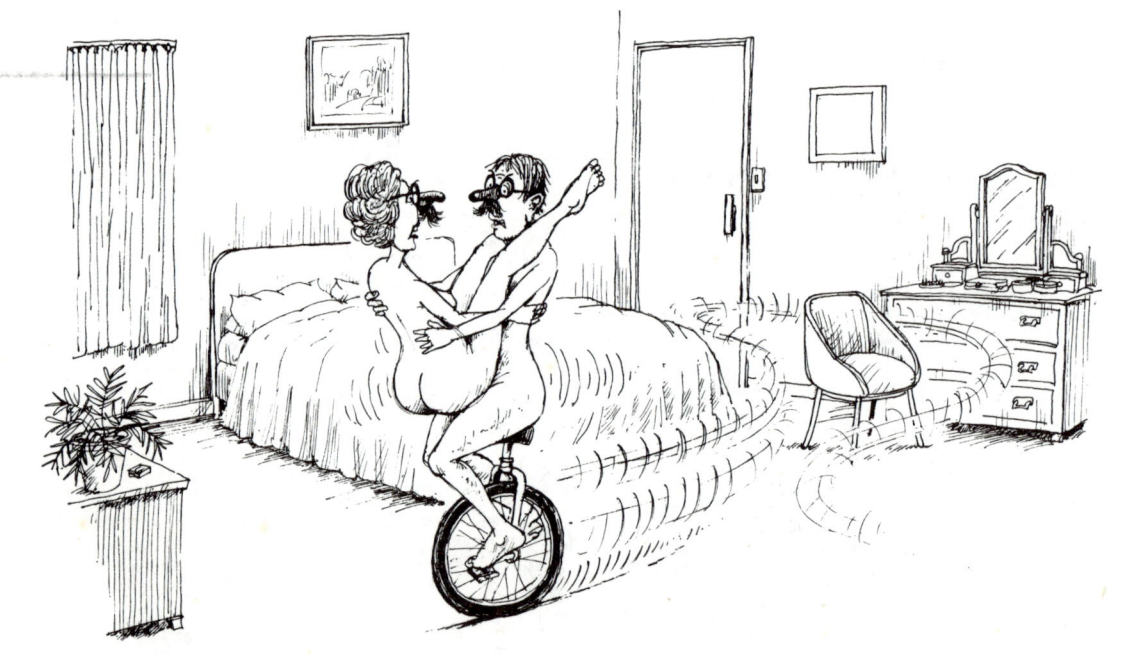

It's no good, Nigel, it just isn't fun any more.